The Light at the Center of Pain

The Light at the Center of Pain

Messages of Hope & Renewal

for People in Chronic Pain

SARAH ANNE SHOCKLEY

Any Road Press

Cover Image: *Resting*, Victor Gabriel Gilbert, 1890

All images public domain, courtesy Wikimedia Commons

ISBN: 978-0-9641279-4-4
Library of Congress: Control Number: 2017906118

Publisher's Cataloging-in- Publication data

Names: Shockley, Sarah Anne, author.
Title: The Light at the center of pain : messages of hope and
renewal for people in chronic pain / Sarah
Anne Shockley.
Description: Fairfax, CA: Any Road Press, 2017.
Identifiers: ISBN 978-0- 9641279-4- 4 | LCCN 2017906118
Subjects: LCSH Chronic pain-- Popular works. | Chronic pain--
Treatment. | Chronic pain-- Alternative
treatment. | Pain-- Popular works. | BISAC HEALTH &
FITNESS / Pain Management
Classification: LCC RB127 .S488 2017 | DDC 616/.0472-- dc23

Praise from Readers...

"I feel like you 'get' me in my pain...Thank you, Sarah, for giving voice to my thoughts, frustrations and hopes as I work through to returning to life."

"Amazing article. I often feel alone in my pain...thank you so much for putting into words the way living with chronic pain makes us feel."

"This is one of the most helpful articles I've read in a long time. Thank you for breaking it down like this."

"It is deeply comforting to know I'm not alone in thinking that I don't know who I am without pain or after it, even though all I want is to be rid of it. Thank you for this."

"This might have been written from the person inside my head who reasons with me when I feel overwhelmed and ruled by pain...It's good to know what I feel is what others feel at times."

"OMG! Exactly what I am going through!...Thank you, we all need to be heard and treated kindly!!!"

"This was absolutely beautiful, articulate, and insightful. Thank you for sharing!"

"Brilliant...adore your wisdoms, your inspirational uplifting words, as well as your survivor mindset!"

"I love that you are choosing to find meaning no matter what the landscape of life looks like...Thank you so much for writing this."

"Great post…I wish I'd been told this 10 years ago."

"Very meaningful…I am going to go back and read it again. Thanks for helping us all through this pain."

"What a refreshing article you have written about living with chronic pain. I really appreciate your sharing the various ways to try to get a better handle on our pain. Many thanks!"

"I think the writing is genius, and I'm definitely going to give it a try. Thank you for this. I hope this helps someone else too."

"Love this …couldn't have said this better…thanks for the articulation!"

"I cannot relate how much I appreciate your column…At least now I know I'm not losing my mind. Thank you!"

"These are great suggestions, and you really hit the nail on the head describing what it's like!...I have to share with my nearest and dearest, hopefully they'll understand a little better!"

"I love that you not only explained what was going on but how to help cope…thank you and keep it up!"

"I am in my 23rd year with neuropathy…Thank you for your insights and your suggestions."

"BEAUTIFUL…I have really enjoyed every post I read here."

To all those seeking to make sense of their pain

DISCLAIMER

Nothing in this book constitutes medical advice and it is not intended to be a substitute for the medical advice of physicians. The reader should consult a physician in matters relating to his or her health and particularly with respect to any symptoms that may require diagnosis or medical attention. The reader understands that they take full responsibility for the effects generated from the use of any suggestions or exercises presented in this book and that it is up to them to use their discretion and common sense in this regard.

CONTENTS

Introduction   ix

1   Life on Planet Pain   1

2   You Can't Be in Pain That Long...Can You?   7

3   When Pain Feels More Real Than You Do   13

4   The Spiritual Practice of Living with Pain   19

5   Giving Pain a Voice   25

6   Are We Really Alone in Our Pain?   33

7   When Practitioners Don't See Our Pain   39

8   Making a Pain Diary Work for You   45

9   Don't Put Your Life on Hold   53

10 The Lone Wolf in Pain   59

11 Staying Visible in the Realms of Pain   65

12 Living with Chronic Pain is a Full Time Job   71

13 Don't Try to Fix Me   77

14 Healing is for the Birds   85

15 Making Our Journey a Thing of Beauty   91

16 Losing and Finding Ourselves in Pain   97

17 The Stories We Tell   103

18 Writing Through Pain to See the Self   111

19 When Magical Thinking is Not Enough   117

20 Truth as a Door to Deep Healing   125

21 Is Pain Pointing Toward Life?   131

22 The Myth of the Holy Grail of Pain   137

23 A Different Kind of Animal   145

24 The Light at the Center of Pain   151

25 Making Peace with Pain   157

    List of Illustrations   163

    About the Author   164

    Other Books by Sarah Anne Shockley   165

INTRODUCTION

This book is a collection of essays based on popular posts from *The Pain Companion Blog*.

The writings are both philosophical and practical in nature–musings, meditations, and advice on living with chronic pain–how it takes over life, how it changes us, how we can better live in response to its demands, and how we can avoid becoming its emotional hostages, and, instead, find a path of greater well being.

I hope you will find emotional solace and understanding here, as well as useful practical support.

I wish you well on your journey through and beyond pain.

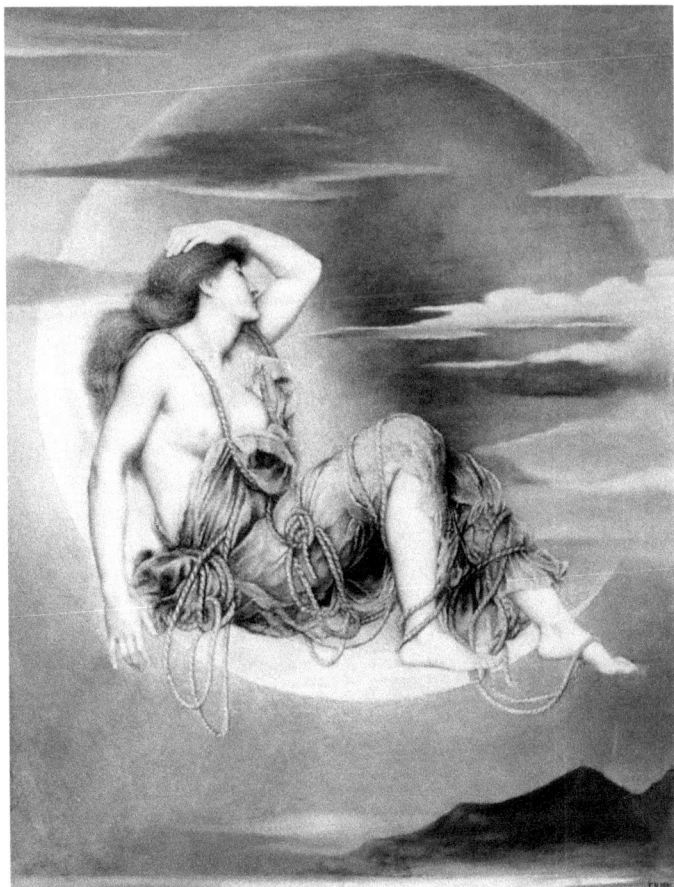

1

Life On Planet Pain

LIVING WITH CHRONIC PAIN is like living on another planet with a completely different atmosphere.

Other pains can usually be pointed to or clearly described. They are polite enough to stay within certain physical or emotional confines, and have a reasonable shelf life.

Chronic pain, on the other hand simply refuses to leave, and often roams around the body wherever it pleases.

To add insult to injury, instead of remaining confined within the physical body, chronic pain sort of oozes out of its original borders and takes over more and more of the territory of our every day experience, eventually seeping through and soaking into the entire fabric of our existence.

Pain Becomes the House We Live In

What was originally on the inside, now feels like its taken over the outside too, as if we are within it, instead of it within us.

At that point, pain isn't just here or there, it's everywhere.

It's really very strange and challenging to explain to others who haven't had the experience. It's like nothing else. Sometimes it feels like an unwanted house guest who never leaves, but eventually it feels like the house itself.

We're surrounded by a field of pain and everything we see, do, hear, express, or receive must pass through the ever-present fog of the pain zone. I think this might be the most difficult thing for others to understand.

Pain is no longer just one aspect of our experience of life, our lives now take place completely immersed within it.

Too Late For A Band-Aid

I think this is one reason it's so hard to find treatments and modalities that actually work for chronic pain. Chronic pain is a complex syndrome which has become interwoven with the entire self and the whole body and the whole nervous system.

Almost everything that is offered to relieve it and to heal it is just too small, or too specialized, or too directed to a single aspect of this all-encompassing thing we know as chronic pain.

It's sort of like the plumber arriving to fix the leak in the kitchen sink when the whole house has just fallen off a cliff.

The well-meaning plumber focuses on the kitchen sink and says, here, let's change the washers or tighten the connections, but we're living in this disaster of a house that needs all kinds of different and simultaneous attentions and the plumber can't see past the broken faucet.

Or something like that.

Looking For The Door That Lets Pain Out

I guess I'm looking for the way off Planet Pain. I imagine it as a door that let's pain out. Like on a spaceship. You open the hatch and everything is sucked into outer space—the whole atmosphere of pain—and then you get to close the door and start over.

It's a nice fantasy, but I suspect that the secret to healing all this pain is less about how to get it out of my body, and more about diving deeply into my inner world and coming to understand its ultimate purpose in the fabric of my whole life.

That the door I'm looking for doesn't open out like that, it opens in.

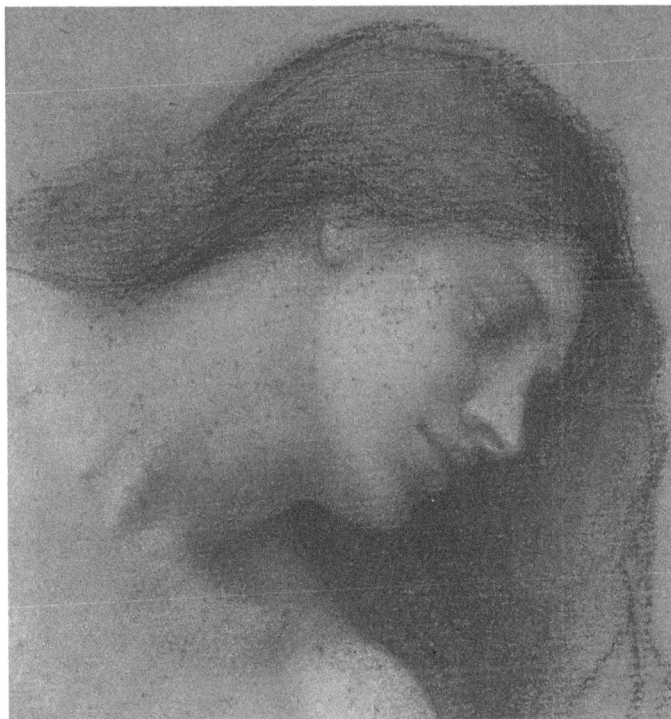

2

You Can't Be In Pain That Long...Can You?

THOSE OF US in chronic pain often have to live with others' inability to accept what's happening with us.

People who aren't in pain often wonder why we aren't better yet. How can anyone be in pain that long, they ask? It's just not *possible*.

Except that we can, and we are, unfortunately. It's real. It's physical. It's tiring, and it demands the utmost of our inner fortitude and emotional stamina to keep going and not sink into a blob of misery on a regular basis.

While we're doing our best to manage our ongoing pain every day, people around us are moving on with their lives. They're moving forward while we, seemingly, are staying in the same place. This can lead to misunderstandings and frustrations on both sides of the experience.

We become frustrated with our pain, with our physical condition, and with ourselves for not healing faster. Others become frustrated with us as well, because we aren't available in the same manner that we used to be. We can't participate or contribute in the ways others are accustomed to us doing, and this can lead to them imagining that we're just not trying hard enough.

Everyone's Got An Idea

We hear, sometimes overtly and sometimes very subtly, that we're probably not doing enough, or we're just not doing the right things. This is often from very well-meaning people, but still...the helpful advice seems to be so often about what we're *not* doing.

We have been told any number of things about why we're still in pain:

- maybe we aren't really working at healing ourselves

- maybe we simply have to try yet another therapy or supplement or magic wand

- maybe we *want* to stay in pain (ouch!)

- maybe our pain is emotionally based (which usually translates into *maybe it's not real*), or another version:

- maybe it's all in our heads (I'm never sure what that really is supposed to mean. Pain is pain. If someone *were* cooking up their physical or emotional pain in their head, then they must be in a lot of pain already at some level to have to do that.)

Pain Turns the World Upside Down

Even some practitioners doubt the possibility of the existence of extreme pain over time, as if the length of time a person is in pain somehow lessens its believe-ability, instead of proving its intensity and intractability.

Yet when others announce that our pain cannot be real, they are dismissing our experience and our reality. It's like saying to us, *you* aren't real.

It's a level of denial, I guess. It's scary to see someone in pain for a long time. It turns the world upside down for people. It's not supposed to happen.

Sometimes it's easier to disbelieve someone who reports experiencing pain for months or years, than it is to admit that relentless, ongoing pain can be a reality...because then it becomes a possibility for anyone, and that might be too much to let in.

And sometimes I think people deny other people's pain so they don't have to look at their own.

How Long Will It Last?

So why does pain stick around so long?

Sometimes we just don't have an answer for that. But because we don't understand how it all works yet, or how to move through it to the other side, doesn't mean it doesn't exist or it isn't real or that we are wrong or mistaken or have failed in some way because we're not all better yet, and are still navigating our way through it.

Is there a far shore without pain for those of us who have lived with it for years? I honestly don't know the answer to that question. I'd like to believe that there is. But I do believe that all of us who must deal with pain on a daily basis are doing it in *exactly the right way for us*, whatever that may be.

This journey is completely individual, there is no one-size-fits-all answer, and, whether anyone else wants to believe it or not, those of us who have lived with chronic pain for any length of time understand that there is no quick and simple answer.

How long will it take to be out of pain? I guess the only answer to that is not a very satisfying one, but it's accurate.

It will take exactly the time that it takes.

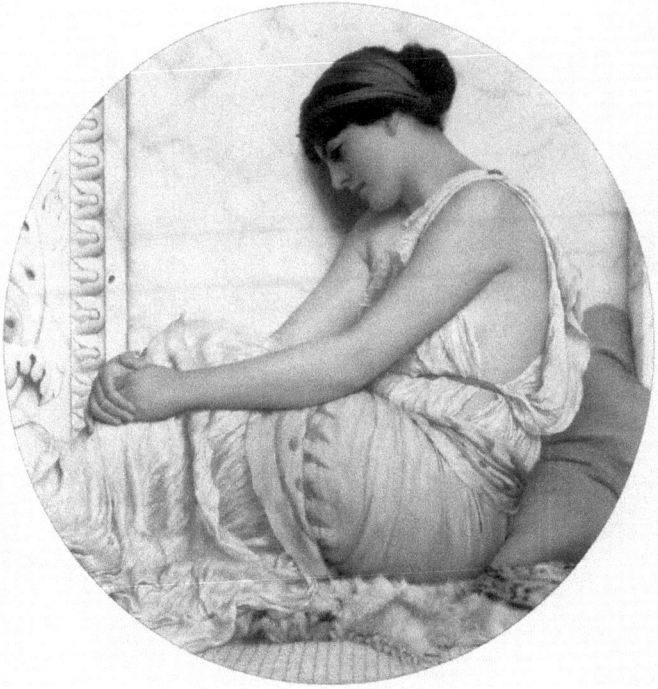

3

When Pain Feels More Real
Than You Do

LIVING WITH PAIN over time, we can feel as if we begin to recede into the background, becoming less and less distinct, like a ghost self in our own life.

Pain takes up more space in our consciousness than many other things, and it takes up a very primary space in our awareness.

We necessarily spend a great deal of time and energy on dealing with our painful condition, treating it, catering to it, and taking it to its appointments and therapies.

Taking a Backseat to Pain

Added to that is the habit we have of speaking about our painful conditions as if they had a life of their own. We talk about *our* pain, *our* condition, *our* symptoms. This is natural, since they are so close to us, so demanding.

But this can feel like we are taking a backseat in life. As if pain were in the driver's seat and our doctor or therapist or pain medication or whatever modality we're using to try and heal ourselves is riding shotgun, and we're relegated to the backseat, hoping we can get a word in edgewise.

It's understandable, but it does feel a bit weird sometimes, that our practitioners seem to have a closer relationship with our pain, our condition, our illness, than they do with us. That's their job, I guess, but it adds to the feeling of being secondary in our own lives.

Which leads to a growing feeling that the pain is becoming more real, and more primary, than we ourselves are.

Reasserting the Self

This is when, despite our low energy and the awfulness of how we're feeling, we need to find a way to reassert ourselves as the primary Center in our own lives.

Pain necessarily demands a lot from us, but we also need to find ways to be ourselves *as* ourselves and *for* ourselves too. Maybe we can only handle doing it in small ways, but that may be enough for now.

Like reading a poem. Or listening to incredibly beautiful music. Or meditating on photos of us in health and just breathing that in. Not as something we have lost, but as something we still are.

Allowing the inner Self the space to express. Making a drawing. Reading something light and funny. Watching comedians on YouTube. Doing something, anything, that reconnects us with us.

And probably on a daily basis. Just one small thing every day. Collecting colorful stones. Buying a flower. Asking someone to bring something beautiful when they visit. Asking them to read to us. Maybe a fairy tale with a happy ending.

I'm Still Here

Is *this* a fairy tale, you may well ask? I'm sick and in pain and you're asking me to find pleasure somewhere? Yes, I guess I am.

Because you're worth re-discovering.

Because, despite pain's apparent primacy, you are still here. And I think it's important to announce that to yourself out loud and with conviction:

I AM STILL HERE.

Because life isn't all about the pain, even if it seems that way sometimes. There is a place, maybe buried under the layers of discomfort, but still, it is there, that is the You of you, and you can touch that place and draw strength from that place.

Will the pain go away if you do that? Maybe, and maybe not, but you will most likely feel better in other ways and that, too, is important.

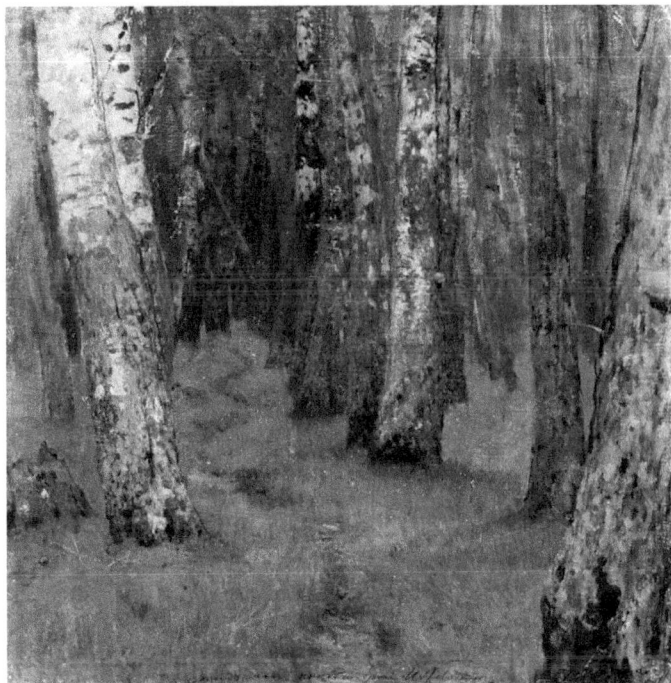

4

The Spiritual Practice of
Living With Pain

FOR MOST OF US, it's pretty difficult to stay cheerful and pleasant when we're in pain and, honestly, I'm not sure it's particularly healthy to try. We do, however, have to keep following the best path we can for ourselves.

We find ways to laugh, to keep a mostly hopeful outlook, and to keep searching for new alternatives and looking out for any light we can perceive in the distance.

Despite our generally positive attitude, however, over time we often find ourselves feeling worn down. We've tried everything to heal our condition and to relieve our pain, yet we're still in it.

A Daily Act of Courage

Sometimes it's easier to fall into a kind of grim resignation than to keep putting energy and hope into treatments and practices that may not seem to be making much of a difference.

Over time, we can sink almost imperceptibly lower and lower emotionally into a kind of ever-present depression, where life seems gray and lifeless and it becomes a major act of courage just to get up and face another day.

I think of this as a kind of seeping loss of hope that can drain whatever remaining well being we have, if we're not careful. Giving up, giving in, abandoning hope, and abandoning ourselves may be just around the corner.

When I feel like this, I have to remind myself that every day I'm alive I'm in some kind of process, or practice. I'm either moving toward more wellness of whatever kind I can manage, physical or emotional, or I am allowing the pain in my body to decide for me how I feel about myself and about life.

If I insist that pain must leave completely before I can be happy again, then I am making *it* the master of my emotional well being.

The Practice of Finding Balance

This effort, to live with pain and not succumb to depression or despondency, is an effort to find emotional, mental, and physical balance within and around the pain–a balance between not forcing myself to be unrealistically bright and cheery, but not wallowing in self pity either. This takes mental and emotional discipline. It becomes a form of daily spiritual practice.

Certainly, living with pain is not a path anyone in their right mind would consciously choose as a spiritual practice for themselves. It is a difficult and lonely path, quiet and internal, and we walk it only out of necessity, but it can also be surprisingly deep and rich.

It's not that being in pain is inherently spiritual, despite the fact that some religions consider suffering to be a holy sacrament (a concept I don't embrace). For me, it's certainly not the suffering or the pain or some kind of sacred martyrdom that gives a spiritual quality to the path through pain. It's how we *are* with the pain. It's what we do and don't do with it and through it.

Standing With The Self Through Pain

For me, the spiritual aspect of the journey isn't that we try to be cheerful or that we think positively or try not to complain and be the perfect patient. In fact, those things can be very counterproductive. For me, it's first and foremost the choice to stay with myself, so to speak, to be true to my own feelings and to learn to stand by me. I am here for *me*.

And that standing with the self, believing in the self, not giving up on the self, whatever that looks like for each of us, can be incredibly hard to do. To not take the way of hating life, of hating who we are, of hating the circumstances–that standing with the self through the difficulties, *is* the path.

23

And when we find the bitterness, the anger, and the hatred rising up–toward ourselves or toward the circumstances–we can feel it and let it pass through. We choose to honor what's coming up, but we choose not to *live* there.

It's a daily spiritual practice to constantly return to openness, to whatever good the day may bring, to be present with ourselves no matter what the circumstances may be, and to express our inner spirits, however little and however much we can manage to do that authentically, despite and through the challenges of living with our pain.

Doing that is a very deep spiritual practice. It takes courage and fortitude, resolution and determination, and an inner choice which we must constantly renew (despite pain's insistence to the contrary) to stick by our true selves, and to remain the center and the heart of our own lives.

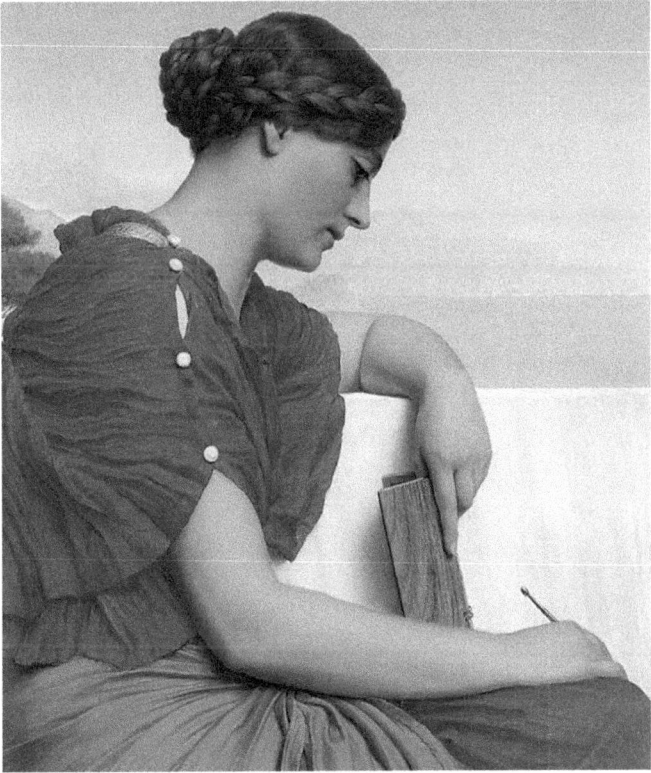

5

Giving Pain a Voice

In ALL THE DISCUSSIONS of how to treat chronic pain with pain meds, various approaches to healing, and alternative treatments and modalities, we don't want to overlook a key aspect of the nature of pain.

Pain is a messenger. It is here because it has something to say. Giving pain a voice can help it, in incremental stages, to complete, release, and move on.

What does it mean to give pain a voice? You may already be familiar with journaling as an excellent way to relieve the emotional ramifications of living with chronic pain, and that's one way to give pain a voice, but I am suggesting something even more direct here.

The Inside Story

Rather than expressing how you feel *about* pain, I'm recommending finding ways to let pain express itself. You could think of it as allowing the part of you that is experiencing physical pain to express from within the pain, and as the pain.

For example: the next time you decide to journal, instead of writing about your own feelings and experiences, try taking a deep breath and stepping into the pain. I know, at first you may think, yuck, why would I step into my pain? It's already hard enough to live with it. But bear with me.

From the experience of being within the pain, begin to write what pain has to say.

Write as if you are your pain speaking. Write about what pain itself feels like to be in your body, what pain wants, what pain is trying to accomplish by being here. Don't try to figure this out in your head. Just go into a slightly altered state of consciousness and let the words flow, even if they seem like nonsense at first.

Ask pain questions, and let it respond. Who are you? What are you? What are you doing in my body? What do you really want? How can I help? How can I soothe? How can I heal?

If it's difficult to step out of your thinking mind and you find yourself trying too hard to come up with answers for pain, try writing with your non-dominant hand.

I Have Something To Say...

The first time you allow pain to express itself may feel a little strange, or silly, or you may come up blank at first. Just be patient. Pain isn't used to being listened to in this way. It might take a moment to register that you actually want to hear what it has to say.

Experiment with other ways to let pain express too. Instead of journaling, you can try speaking for pain. Designate a chair in the room as pain's chair for the time being.

Then go sit in it and speak into the room as pain (or do this from bed if you aren't mobile right now). Just let the words flow.

Pain may surprise you. It may express as very angry about being stifled all the time. Or very tender. Or confused. Or incredibly sad.

Don't try to analyze it while it's happening. Just let pain express as pain wants to, however that is. Right now, even though pain feels like a nasty invader, it's living in your body and it's a part of your experience that needs to be heard.

It's a part of you that is expressing *as* pain.

Humming, Vocalizing, Singing, Lamenting

Another method is to use your voice to express pain as a sound. (You might want to wait until you're alone for this one.) Take a breath and go into the experience of pain in your body, and then begin to hum from that place.

Experiment with very high and very low pitches. Let the hum express the sound of pain. Just let it come out. Soft, loud, plaintive, or angry.

Then, if you're feeling adventurous, let the humming morph into other sounds: moans, groans, high pitched whines, sobs, sighs. Whatever sounds want to come from the pain in your body. It's most freeing to let go of your expectations of what sounds pain might make, and just let the noises come out in whatever form they want to take.

If you're self conscious or there are others in the house you don't wish to disturb, you can make noises into a pillow. Just make sure *you're* listening. You are the most important person to hear the sounds of your own pain. It is a way of witnessing, validating, and releasing the pain you're in.

If you're musically inclined, you might want to make up a song of lament, or a song of freedom. Give pain center stage and full voice for as long as it takes to feel a sense of release.

It All Helps

This practice may strike you as naively over simplified, but I have found throughout my pain journey that the most potent remedies for ongoing pain are very, very straightforward and simple.

Resting often. Reducing stress and staying as calm as possible. Releasing held or restricted breath and allowing its life-giving and healing force to move more freely through the body.

And giving pain a voice.

Remember, no single thing you do to heal, soothe, express, or release your pain is going to be the whole story of your healing. Yet all of the simple, yet profound practices we put into effect on a daily basis have a positive cumulative effect. I can testify to that.

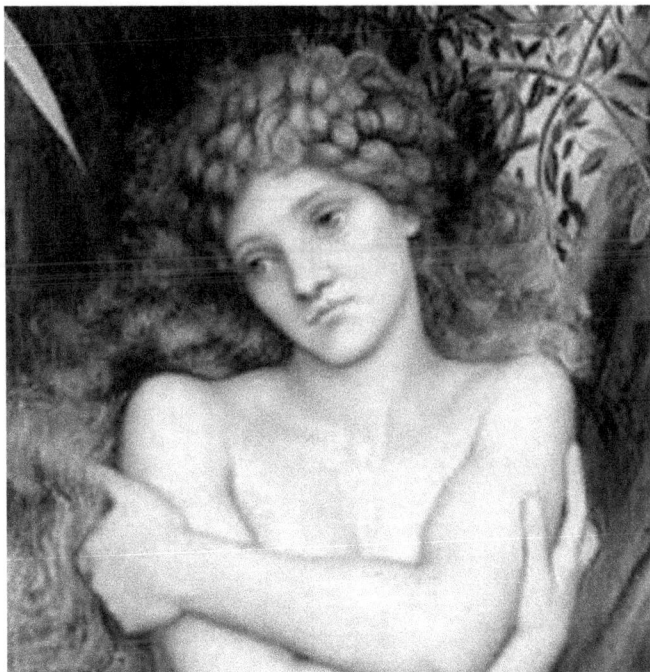

6

Are We Really Alone in Our Pain?

EVERYONE WHO HAS BEEN in pain for some length of time has asked themselves these questions: *Why is this happening to me? What did I do wrong to deserve this?*

We struggle with feelings of guilt and shame for needing help, for not being able to fix ourselves, for probably asking too much of everyone around us, for causing people to feel bad for us, for needing financial assistance.

Just Try Harder...

Some pain comes in and won't leave. There may not be a tidy explanation, but it doesn't mean that we are off our center, or we are lacking in some fundamental way, or we are not good people, or not in alignment with God or the Universe, or that we haven't prayed or fasted or meditated enough, or burnt off our karma yet. Being in pain does not automatically put you at fault.

The fact that you don't have an off switch for your pain does not mean that you aren't trying hard enough or that in some insidious way you must want to be in pain. It does not mean that you have failed, or were probably a terrible person in a past life.

Asking Different Questions

Being in pain doesn't prove anything negative about you at all. An estimated 1 in 3 Americans are in pain right this moment. That's a lot of people.

So, the questions we might want to begin to ask about all this pain may be more about ourselves as a culture rather than ourselves as individuals.

Yes, we may ask ourselves, *What can I do differently in my life to relieve this pain?*, but we also may need to ask, *How are we, as a people, creating so much pain for ourselves?* Then the answers become less of a private struggle and more of a community effort toward greater harmony and balance at all levels of our lives.

And if this epidemic of pain is as much of a collective as a private experience, then maybe part of the solution is to understand that we are, somehow, all in this together.

That the healing needed may not only be along a solitary path, but something we need to address as a society. We have somehow created a culture where violence and alienation is the norm and, perhaps our painful bodies go hand in hand with that.

Is it remotely possible that some of us may be feeling our collective alienation from the earth and from each other as illness and pain in our bodies?

And This Helps Me How?

You might well ask, how does speculating about this help me with my pain today?

For me, as much as I would not want to wish this experience of pain on anyone, it eases my mind to know that I'm not alone in it, that there seems to be something bigger at work here than my own private path through it, and that, while the answer may not be easy, it may also not be entirely up to me to figure it out all on my own. And, right now, today, that is something of a comfort.

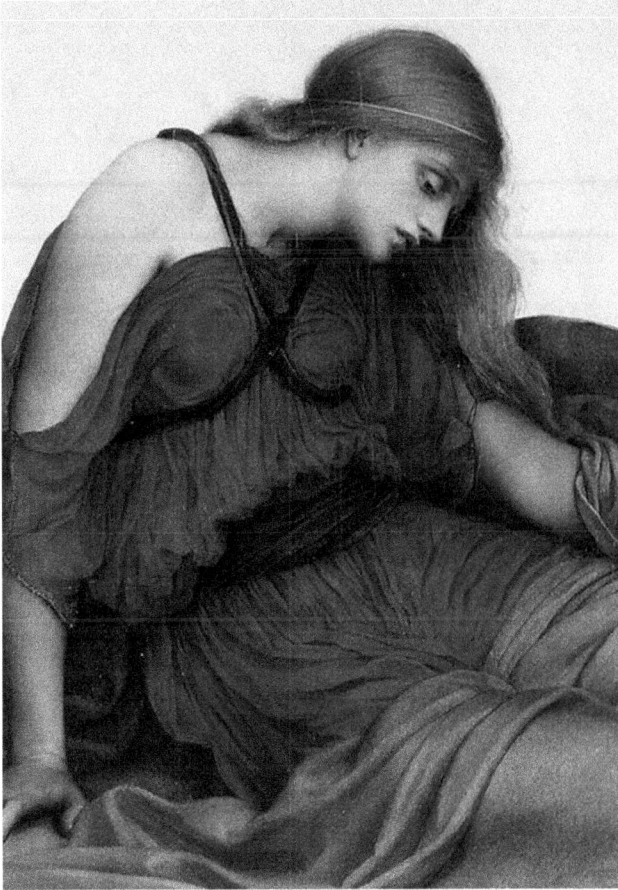

7

When Practitioners Don't

See Our Pain

ONE OF THE MOST challenging situations for those of us in chronic pain is when we are working with a medical or therapeutic practitioner who is unable to see or understand the intensity of our suffering. They may also feel that its longevity is either questionable or somehow due to something we, as patients, are not doing right.

Sometimes we are told to do things that are painful for us, yet are not believed when we report that it hurts. Sometimes we are told that we simply can't be in the pain we're in. Practitioners have made a career of helping people in pain, yet when they invalidate clients' experiences, they inadvertently cause more pain.

How does this happen? How do highly trained, and very caring, individuals end up causing more pain for the patients they are trying to cure?

Not Feeling Heard

This can manifest in a number of ways:

- A treatment or protocol isn't working, or is causing more pain, but the practitioner insists that we continue or try harder, because they believe in the treatment more than in our feedback.

- The practitioner may have experience working with people in pain, but has never had to live with chronic pain themselves, so does not understand the difference between short-term pain and long-term pain. They do not understand the side effects of chronic pain, which can include loss of brain power, fatigue, fogginess, and sleep deprivation, and simply don't take these into account.

- The practitioner does not believe that our particular condition causes the level of pain we are in, and works with us as if we have a different version of that condition or a different condition altogether.

- They have an intense desire to help and would rather believe that we are wrong than admit that they are unable to offer us a cure.

As a client, this is very difficult to deal with. It makes us feel unheard, misunderstood, and belittled. Not to mention the fact that we may feel shamed for not healing as fast as we're *supposed* to or for not responding to treatment in the same way the norm does.

This is not to say that there aren't any medical

practitioners who listen to their clients. There are many caring, compassionate, and sensitive practitioners who listen and take note of what their clients report and adjust their treatments and recommendations accordingly. But, unfortunately, there are also many who don't listen. Or they listen, but they discount what they hear.

For these practitioners, unfortunately, the fact that the treatment they are offering isn't working doesn't always indicate to them that they need to find different ways of handling chronic pain. For some of them, it's easier to blame the patient.

Your Expertise Versus My Expertise

It's important to learn to speak up for ourselves. However, when we're in pain, it can be very challenging to take a stand of any kind. We're usually exhausted and operating on limited brainpower.

Often it's difficult to do anything more than barely stumble through a medical appointment. Despite this, I do feel that it is up to those of us who live with chronic pain to educate the medical establishment when we have the opportunity to do so.

I have written some talking points to help you begin the conversation with your practitioner, if you choose to.

- *I respect you as an expert in your field. I ask you to*

respect me as an expert in how I am experiencing pain in my own body.

- *When you insist that you know more about my experience of pain than I do, I feel belittled and invalidated.*

- *My direct experience is the most valid basis we have to assess how treatments are working or not working, and I ask you to be willing to listen to my feedback and take it into account.*

- *If treatments do not work for me in the same way that they do for the majority of your patients, it does not mean I am not trying hard enough. It does not give you a basis for discounting my experience. It means there is something new to learn here.*

One thing that can be very helpful is to keep a pain diary, a record of the kind and level of pain you experience from day to day, and bring it with you to medical appointments. (See the following section, *Making A Pain Diary Work For You.*)

It's too bad that those of us who are already in pain sometimes have to endure more pain, both physical and emotional, when we're working with certain practitioners. I wish it were not so.

However, I believe, that since some practitioners seem ill equipped to work with long-term pain, it may be up to us to educate them with our gentle, but insistent truth.

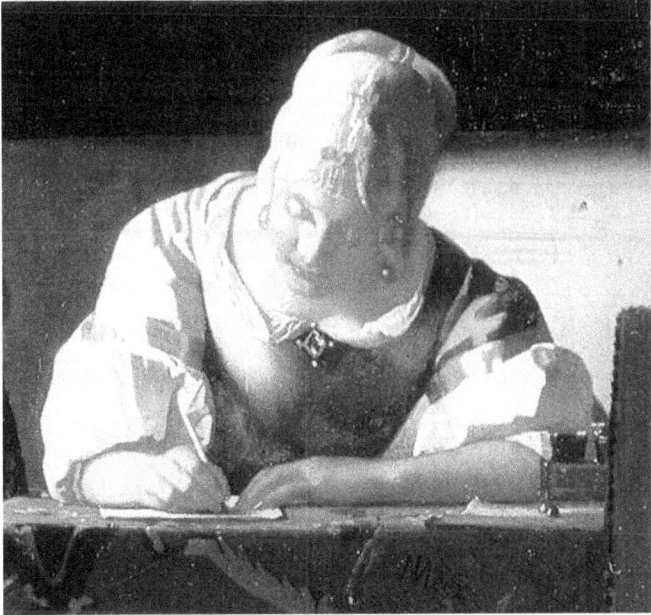

8

Making A Pain Diary Work For You

A PAIN DIARY is a daily record you keep for yourself detailing the nature and levels of the physical or emotional pain you are experiencing.

Why would you want to keep a record of your pain? Tracking your pain sounds like one of the least appealing things you could do.

Yes, I know, but there are a number of reasons why it can be very helpful for chronic pain sufferers to do so. Read on.

Why Keep A Pain Diary?

Here are some valuable reasons for making the effort to monitor and record your pain experience:

- To provide credibility about the nature and level of your specific pain(s) which you can show to medical practitioners and therapists, particularly if they have difficulty understanding the intensity or duration of your pain.

- To provide important details for your physician about how your medication is working or not working, and any side effects.

- A pain diary can be helpful to share with caregivers so that they can better understand your needs.

- Tracking your pain levels helps you see when your pain tends to be most intense so that you can plan rest, appointments, and work accordingly (at least as much as is possible).

- A pain diary helps you more clearly see which activities affect your pain levels for good or ill.

- Sometimes these records can be useful for insurance or legal purposes.

Okay, you say, I can see some of the uses for a pain diary, but how do I go about creating one that's easy to keep, easy to refer to, and actually useful?

How To Set Up Your Pain Diary

Here are some simple guidelines that have worked for me.

- Plan to keep the diary for at least one week, but longer is highly recommended if you're up for it (since tracking pain over a longer time span provides more information).

- Use a small notebook that's easy on your hands and a felt tip pen or other writing utensil that's easy to use and writes clearly.

- At the top of each page write the date.

- In the first notes of the day, jot down how much sleep you think you got and the quality of sleep: Did you sleep fitfully, soundly, or not at all? Did you get up in the night?

- Make notes on pain at least 4 times a day, if at all possible (upon waking, mid-day, afternoon, and evening), noting specific times.

- At each check-in time, note your overall level of discomfort, and then any specific pains and their levels, noting changes in pain quality or intensity. Use the 1–10 pain scale, since practitioners tend to prefer it, but also use descriptive words. If things are pretty much the same, just write *Same*.

Keep It Clear And Simple

If you only have energy for the minimum of 4 check-ins a day, do that.

For a more complete diary, and if you want to track the efficacy (and side effects) of medication and/or the effects of physical therapy protocols, then I suggest adding the following into your daily notes as well:

- Medications taken and at what times.

- Any exercise and physical therapy you do, the

time you did them, and duration.

- Note periods of rest.

- Keep it simple so that doing this does not become a burden. These are notes, rather than an old-fashioned Dear Diary description of everything you do and feel. (I recommend a separate Pain Journal if you wish to go more deeply into what you're feeling and experiencing on a deep emotional level.)

- Use phrases instead of full sentences.

- Use highly descriptive words (see suggested list below).

- Use the 1–10 scale consistently, and in a way that makes sense to you so that you can easily communicate it to others.

Sounds like a lot, but you can use shorthand. For example, if you have a regular routine of physical therapy exercises you do, just write PT and the time. No need for further details unless the routine significantly increases or decreases your pain.

The following lists of descriptive words are offered to make it easier for you to express yourself and help you find the words you need. The lists are not meant to be exhaustive, but I hope they show that descriptive words communicate much more clearly to others than the words "pain" or "hurt" do by themselves.

Physical Pain:

sharp, dull, twinge, sting, shooting pain, tender, irritated, raw, spasm, pulling, cramping, needle-like, achy, stabbing, throbbing, burning, numb, tingly, tight, sore, queasy, flu-like, dizzy, fatigued, exhausted, listless, light, deep, intense, excruciating, brain fog, easing, releasing, letting up.

Emotional Pain:

low, depressed, angry, despondent, frustrated, hopeless, hopeful, numb, scared, terrified, anxious, confused, stuck, sad, lonely, isolated, ashamed, resentful, sinking, uplifted, tense, relaxed, relieved.

If you are keeping a Pain Diary primarily of your physical pain, it's up to you whether or not you want to add your emotional state into your notes and how comfortable you feel sharing that with others.

Remind Me Why I'm Doing This

Why not just explain all this verbally the next time you see your doctor? Mostly because our brain in pain doesn't work well: we often can't remember details, the right words don't come easily, we're exhausted, we can't think straight, and we used up all our available energy just getting to the appointment.

If the Pain Diary sounds challenging to set up, you're welcome to download a free Pain Diary template at www.thepaincompanion.com on the Resources page, then print it out and write on it or use it as a basis for your own diary and modify as needed.

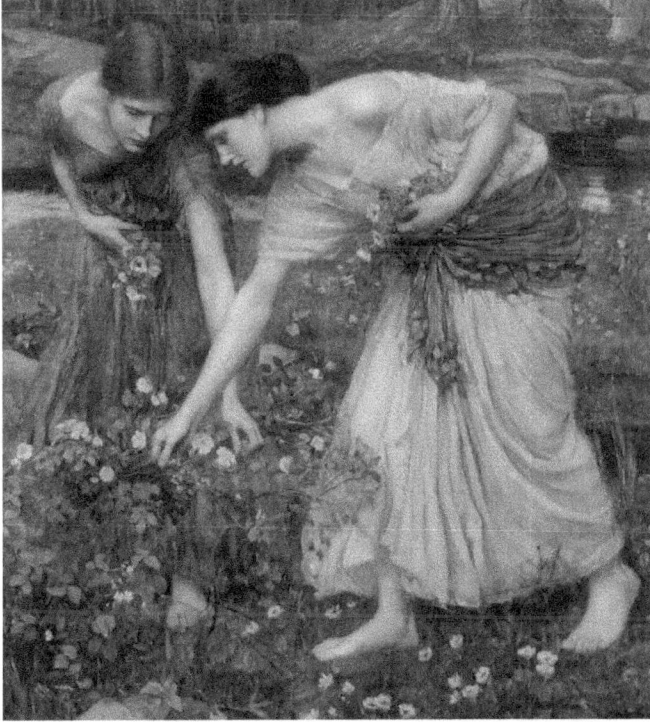

9

Don't Put Your Life on Hold

CONSCIOUSLY OR UNCONSCIOUSLY, we tend to put our "real" life on hold when we're in deep emotional or physical pain.

We think we just have to get through this thing, this phase, this difficulty, and then we will return to our lives when it will be all right to re-engage and participate again.

Of course, there are activities we necessarily have to stop doing when we're in deep pain, that goes without saying. But, in addition to the restrictions that come with our specific condition, we sometimes stop participating with others almost entirely, and, in that way, put our lives on hold.

Re-Including Ourselves

There can be times for non-participation as part of the path through pain. We may feel we have to withdraw from others for a time in order to heal. We need more rest and less stimulation than normal, and we often need to pull away from group situations in order to give ourselves that space.

But it's also important to find ways to step back into life, to re-include activities we enjoy and people we enjoy, in whatever capacity we can, even while we are still living with pain.

When we're in pain, we may not remember that we are still important to others. We still have an impact on the people who love us. They miss being with us, they still care for us, and they are part of our overall connection with life.

When we feel terrible, it's easy to forget that we are still lovable and still loved. Withdrawing because we assume that people don't want us around, or because we can't participate fully, cuts off opportunities for loving engagement with life. It's not entirely healthy, and it's often not a very happy situation either.

Allowing Love

We can find online communities of others who are on this path through pain and these are very important and valuable places to go to feel fully seen, heard and understood, but we also want to be careful that we don't create an exclusive club of people in pain only. While we do have to adjust our lives to accommodate our current limitations, we don't want to narrow them down so much that we lose our connection with its ongoing flow.

When we're in pain for a long time, it's true, some of our friends and acquaintances will no longer be part of our lives, they will move on without us. But others will want to stay connected. I think it's important to find out who is still there for us, who tries to understand, who tries to hear, who offers to help in whatever way they can.

And it's important to reach out, not just for help (which is, in itself, a very important movement), but to reach toward life itself and toward engagement—not to wait for the pain to stop before we carry on with life.

We may not be able to be with others or participate in life in the same capacity as before, nevertheless, our ability to love is still present and we must never allow that to be shut down completely by pain. When we withdraw fully from life, we aren't being abandoned by others, we are the ones who are pulling away.

More Than Getting Through

While we're working through our pain, it's so important to continue to find ways to reach out in love, and to express love. To let dear ones know that, even in pain, we care about them. No loving gesture is too small. A phone call, an email, a cup of tea, a short visit, a meet-up, an update. *I'm still here. I still love you.*

We may choose to put our life on hold while we're in pain, but it doesn't wait for us. It keeps flowing on.

That can become a great sadness if we wake up a few years later and realize we've disconnected ourselves from the mainstream, from our friends, and even from our family.

It's sad, and it's frightening. It's best to find ways, however small, to remain connected with others and connected with life, even as we're on this challenging and often lonely journey through pain.

Especially while we're on this challenging and lonely journey.

As the oft-quoted musician, Prince, once stated, "Dearly Beloved, we are gathered here today to get through this thing called life." We are *all* gathered here. This earth is too small for any of us to pull away into our own solo paths of sorrow and suffering. We're all in it together. And, hopefully, we can not just get through it, but find new ways to thrive, to flourish, to create, to love, and to dream.

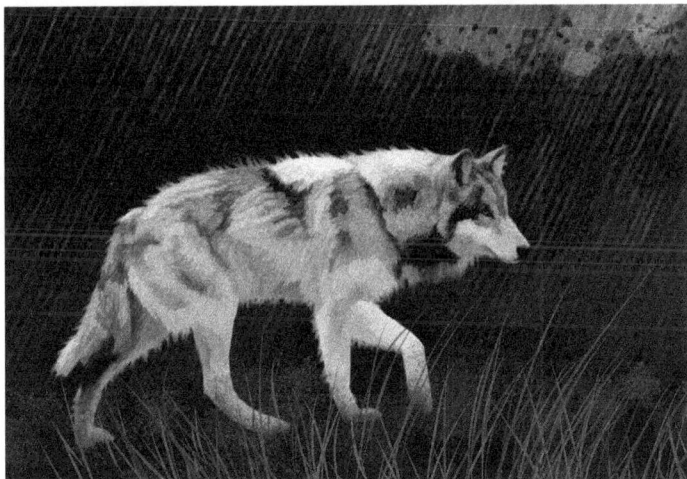

10

The Lone Wolf in Pain

SOME OF US in chronic pain have spent our lives living as lone wolves. We're very resourceful and independent, we don't ask a lot of others, and we tend to be fairly comfortable with being alone.

It comes naturally to us to take care of ourselves, and not be a burden to those around us. We don't rely on others in order to be okay with ourselves. All that is well and good until–

–we get injured or fall ill or have an operation, and find ourselves in ongoing pain, functioning at a much lower capacity than we are used to.

Being Weak is Not Who We Are

And that's not just hard on our bodies, it's hard on our identity and our way of being.

When we have to ask for support, whether financial or emotional, or we can't do all the things we used to be able to do easily we feel as if we our failing–failing others, and failing ourselves.

We believe in independence and self reliance. We subscribe to the DIY attitude toward everything, including healing. We want to make everything work out right now, today. So we may perceive our pain and vulnerability as a weakness–and that feels both terrifying and intolerable.

It's very hard, it's incredibly frustrating, and it can be very scary when you've been used to being the one upon whom others rely for support, for constancy, for dependability, and now you can't fully rely on yourself or your body.

I'll Handle This On My Own, Thanks

And when we're in pain, we want to revert to our lone wolf mode, because it's the most natural thing for us.

We pull away and withdraw from others to lick our wounds alone–to heal by ourselves. We try to cover up the degree of pain we are in, we don't ask for much help, and we keep going as if we are not actually in terrific pain.

But pulling away and going solo isn't always helpful in this case.

Because no one can really understand what we're going through if we don't share with them.

Because if we don't ask, how will people know we need help?

Because if we don't admit we need that help–even to ourselves–we will over do it, strain ourselves, and possibly create more pain.

Because not letting others be there for us sends a message that we don't trust them, and it cuts us off from loving support – both emotional and physical.

So, as unnatural as it may feel for some of us, we might want to do something a little radical, a little uncomfortable. We might want to consider adopting more of a pack mentality, if only for the time we're in pain.

Just This Once...

In a pack, even a small one, we can find solace from sharing our story, and listening to others who have had or are having similar experiences.

We may find we have something beautiful and resourceful and insightful to offer when we open up and allow ourselves to express the pain we're in and how it has affected us.

We learn that asking for help is not always a burden, and that others sometimes find meaning in being there for us.

We find increased health benefits from the greater emotional well being we can gain from finding a pack that includes us, instead of excluding ourselves from the company and support of others.

If we can release our lone wolf mentality just a little–

release the belief that we *have* to go through it alone–do it alone–find our way alone–we can discover that that there not only is there a community, there are helping hands, there are common experiences.

We may discover that accepting some help now and then doesn't mean we're weak, it means we're connected–and that is always a strength.

And when we're out of pain, we can always go back to being the lone wolf again, of course–if we still want to.

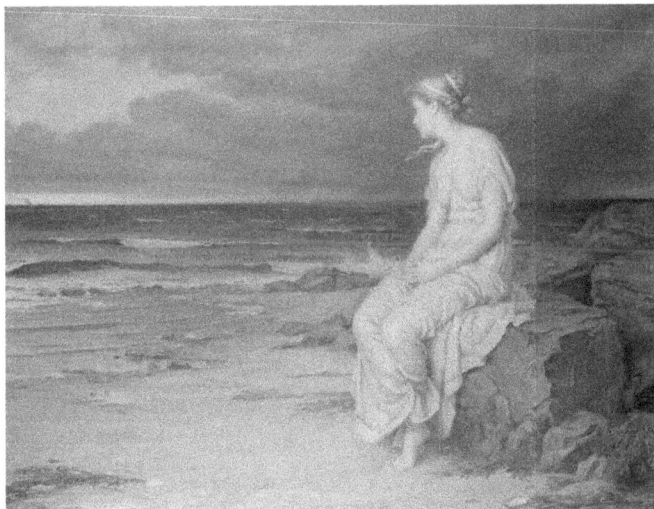

11

Staying Visible In
The Realms Of Pain

SOMETIMES PEOPLE who aren't in pain imagine that those of us who are must have done something wrong.

The exact wrong thing we did is a bit unclear, but it must certainly exist and it is something they would never do. As if there's a clear sign in the road: *No Pain–Go Left. Pain–Go Right.* (Thinking that helps them feel safe–if there is something concrete that we have done wrong to be in so much pain, then surely they can avoid it and it will never happen to them.)

In the Land of Pain

There isn't a sign. Or at least not one that any of us in chronic pain was able to read in time. It's more like the floor drops out from under you, and there you are in the Land of Pain. I write my books and blog to try and make sense of my own sudden and unplanned detour here.

I wrote because I was drowning. I was drowning in physical pain with no end in sight. I looked around my tiny house and it seemed that my whole life had shrunk to that Lilliputian size.

I had given up almost everything because my

condition demanded it. I had contracted my life, shrunk down within it, and withdrawn from just about everything out of necessity since almost every activity other than walking made my pain worse.

I sat in my little cottage and felt the fear of disappearing forever inside my own house of pain. *I can't let this happen*, I thought. *I cannot become this pain.* And yet, it seemed that in many ways I already had. Pain and my physical infirmity dictated everything about my life.

I was losing myself.

No Known Exit Code

Pain had become the air I breathed, the ground I walked on. Pain was both the prison and the guard. If you have been in pain for any length of time, you know what I mean.

Changing our attitude toward pain might make the cell a little more comfortable, but it doesn't necessarily provide the key to the cell door. There is a secret exit code that nobody seems to know, but which cannot be bypassed.

Some people have said to me *Oh, how great to have all that free time!* Um. No. If you have a body that works well and isn't in pain, more time to do nothing would doubtless be a blessing. But all that "free time" in which to sit or lie or walk slowly in intense pain...not so much.

So, I write. I write to throw a voice out from the submerged world of pain. Not to bring more pain out into the world, but to allow myself a way to reconnect, to feel less invisible, to cast a line out from the depths. To maintain some kind of presence in life. To stay visible while living in the realms of pain. Visible to others, and visible to myself.

If the line I throw out catches somewhere, or if someone connects with it, maybe I can use it to haul myself back up and out again, because there is no obvious ladder out of the inner wells of chronic pain.

Staying Visible

Those of us in persistent pain sometimes keep ourselves small and silent so we won't infect the world, thinking that if we speak it can only be with the voice of pain, and therefore will only create more.

So, we figure it's best to remain silent. Remain unseen. It's as if we feel we can't re-enter the world fully until we are pain free.

But we must find ways to re-include ourselves in the world somehow right now. Maybe only in small ways at first, and according to our physical limitations.

We are a community within a community, the

community of people in constant pain, but we are also part of the collective, and it is important to give voice to our experiences both to remain an active part of our collective experience *and* to enrich it.

We must not let the invisibility of our pain become the invisibility of ourselves.

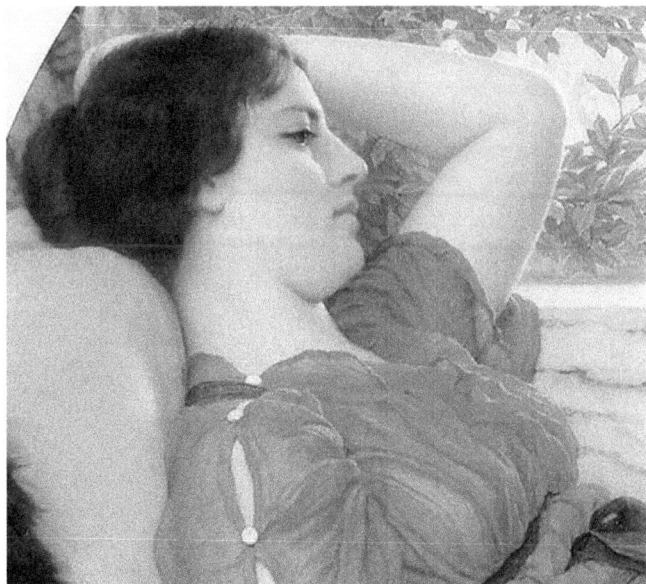

12

Living With Chronic Pain
Is A Full Time Job

WE USUALLY THINK of side effects as the negative by-products of ingesting pharmaceuticals, but chronic pain produces its own side effects.

These side effects result from the many challenges of living with pain that go far beyond the experience of the pain itself.

Experiencing any of them can be distressing, especially if we don't realize that other people are having them too.

All That From Pain?

Side effects from chronic pain include a myriad of emotional and physical challenges. One that can be the hardest to explain to others not experiencing pain, and which can create the most self blame and misunderstanding I call: It Takes All Day To Do (Almost) Nothing.

When we're in constant pain, it can literally take most of our day to get out of bed, wash up, get dressed, eat something, and make a cup of tea. If we're having a good day, maybe we can make one important phone call or complete one page of a form before we're done.

Why is this important to recognize? Because too often we think we are supposed to continue keeping everything together *despite* our pain. We think we're supposed to buck up, be strong, and just keep going.

Why doesn't it work that way? Because just *being* in pain takes most of our energy. End of story.

Today, I Give Myself A Pass

We don't get much done in a day because being in chronic pain *is* what we're doing all day.

When we're in pain our experience of time is different. Our experience of energy and what we can do with it is different. Our entire consciousness is different. We are living in a different world with very different parameters, limitations and no meaningful timetable.

It's important that we recognize this fact and give ourselves a break and stop expecting so much. We can't keep up with life as usual. We probably can't keep up with even a fraction of what we used to do.

We need to give ourselves permission to unhook, unplug, de-stress, and move very slowly, AND we need to gently inform the significant others in our lives of these facts.

So what do we do about this? Take an online course for increasing productivity? NO! Read a bestseller on doing more with less? NO!

The very simple and important answer is: *we live within our present limitations.*

I know it's very hard to not feel guilty about doing very, very little, especially if we are Type A individuals or are parenting in pain. Or both. We worry about losing ground or not being there for our kids, I know.

But chronic pain is something that can't be muscled through. Persistent pain takes up most of who we.

Beating ourselves up emotionally because we can't do as much as we used to do is not going to help us get through this faster or in a more healthful way. We're only adding to the pain we're already in.

Healing Is A Full Time Occupation

So, as much as is possible, it's important to understand that our current occupation is healing. We need to let ourselves off the hook as often as we can and honor our current physical restrictions.

The reason we're not doing much is not because we're lazy, or we're taking advantage of other people, or we're letting pain take over, or we're failing to heal. We're doing very little because our body is putting most of its energy into healing.

Even though we may hate the fact that we're unable to do much while in pain, our limitations are good for us. They force us to slow down, breathe, stop trying so hard, relax, and focus mostly on doing whatever we need to do to heal. Even if it means that sometimes it takes all day to have a cup of tea.

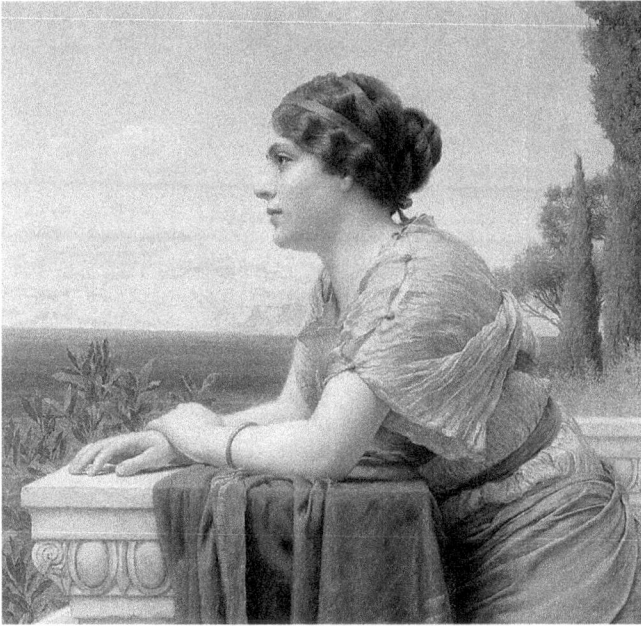

13

Don't Try To Fix Me

I CAN'T TELL YOU how many times some random person has offered unasked-for advice on ending my chronic pain, or a professional healer I just barely met in a social setting has assured me (the minute they find out I have a physical challenge) that they can make me pain free.

Has this happened to you? It just happened again for the umpteenth time yesterday, so I felt I wanted to address it here.

We Appreciate Your Concern, But...

Here's what I'd like to say to these loving, but misguided people on behalf of those of us in chronic pain:

Thank you so much for caring. Truly.

We respect and honor that you really want to help us get better, and that you may even be experts in your field. Please respect and honor that we are also experts—experts in living with our specific conditions and pains.

You probably don't know that we get people telling us how to heal ourselves all the time. And that puts

79

us in the position of having to constantly say no, of having to justify not taking all of that advice or hiring all those healers who want to massage, balance, or re-align us or fill us full of some miracle supplement.

It puts us in the position, over and over again, of looking like we're not trying hard enough, we're not willing to listen, we're, in short, made wrong over and over again by your insistent offers of advice.

How Can I Put This?

We understand your sincerity and your very real eagerness to help, and we don't want to just blow you off, so we feel we have to explain ourselves to you.

We tell you about all the things we've already done, how chronic pain is different and not that simple, not so easy to deal with.

This puts us in the very strange and uncomfortable position of constantly having to defend the pain we're in, which is a really unpleasant feeling, and not one we enjoy.

Can you imagine? You're walking around with a broken leg in a cast and people keep coming up to you and giving you advice for how to treat smelly feet or what to do for a hangnail!

You have to keep explaining over and over again that a broken leg is much worse than that, it takes a lot longer to heal, you're already doing everything you know how to do, and, thanks very much, but that advice isn't really applicable.

Can you imagine how exhausting that would be, especially if the person offering the hangnail treatment is insulted that you aren't as excited about it as they are?

Curb Your Enthusiasm

As healing professionals, when you start the conversation by telling us that we shouldn't be or no longer have to be in pain (presumably because you've turned up), you're unwittingly making us wrong for still experiencing pain, and putting yourself in the position of savior.

I'm sure it's entirely unintentional, but it's kind of an insult to our intelligence and motivations, and minimizes the incredible challenges inherent in actually coming out the other side of pain permanently. You've implied that being in pain is wrong, therefore we're wrong, and you're going to set us right.

Being in pain is not where we want to be, but it is also not a deficiency of character.

If we could be out of pain, we would. We are not resisting healing. We are in chronic pain.

Maybe Try This Instead

Here's what we would most prefer you do when we meet:

First, if we haven't purposefully sought out you or your advice, ask our permission to talk with us about our chronic pain. Please don't start the conversation by telling us what we should be doing.

Second, if we're open to talking about it, find out what our specific condition is, how it affects us (don't assume you know), how extensive it is, how long we've had it, and what we've done already.

Third, if you still feel you have something to offer, ask our permission to present whatever piece of advice or healing modality that may be. Please don't be offended if we simply say, thanks, but no thanks.

Fourth, be honest. If you've helped other people, great, we may want to hear about it, but don't make wild claims about how you can heal us almost instantly when no one else has. Chronic pain is complex and long term, that's why it's *chronic*, it doesn't lend itself to quick fixes.

Fifth, be gracious if, after hearing what you have to say, we decline to work with you or take your advice. Please don't assume that it means that we don't want to heal.

I'm sure you believe that your method or supplement or diet or exercise is *the* right one, but so does everyone else. Pushing it on us makes us as uncomfortable as someone pushing their religious beliefs on us. We can make up our own minds, thanks.

Thanks For Not Sharing

If we decide to work with you and take your advice, know that it will be one layer of a multi-layered approach to healing. This means that it is unlikely that any one thing will completely heal our chronic condition, including the one approach you are offering.

It's a many-layered, long-term effort. Don't keep asking us if we're all better now. And if we don't improve, or if we get worse, let's agree that it's not your fault, and it's not ours either.

In summary, know that we appreciate your caring, but please give us a break with all the advice. Don't feel bad if we decline to call your favorite massage therapist or book a session with you as a healer. We're already working full time on healing.

Thank you for your concern. Really. And the best advice we can give *you* in regard to offering your services or advice? Wait until we ask for it.

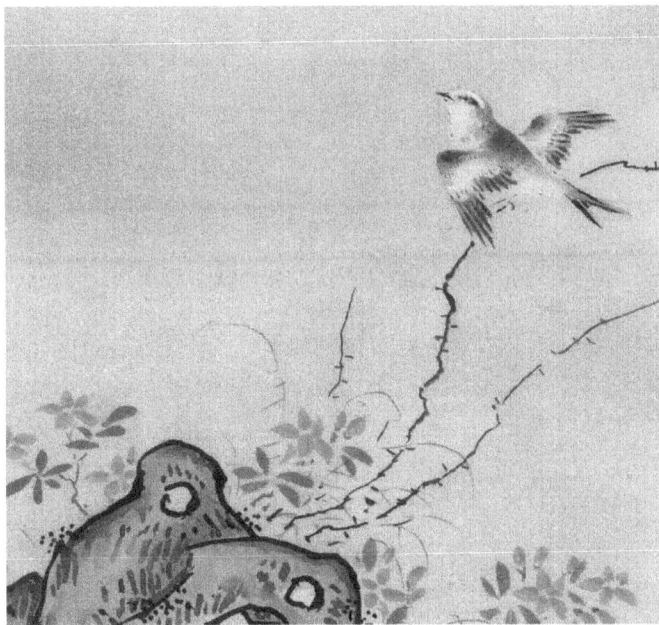

14

Healing Is For The Birds

THIS MORNING I was walking in my neighborhood and stopped to admire the vista from one of the few undeveloped lots. It's a steep grassy hillside that slopes down away from the road and provides a view of trees, hills and houses in the distance.

Several swallows flitted and swooped back and forth in circles close to the grass, catching bugs, I assumed. As I stood there admiring the swallows' flight, one of them flew in slow circles closer and closer to me.

Included In a New Way

Finally, it swooped around me, including me in its flight range. It didn't feel like it was trying to chase me away, instead, it just felt friendly. The swallow dipped back down to the grassy area and then up and around just behind me again and again for several minutes, making large, graceful circles around me.

I just stood there, breathing quietly and enjoying the playful attention. I realized that I had not been completely still in Nature and just watched it and enjoyed it for a long time. I was usually walking through it or driving past it, but not stopping to just *be* in it.

I watched the easy, graceful flight, the joyful turns and flutters and soaring movements of the birds for a few minutes. I could see the gray wings and the patterns of blue and white on their little backs. I noticed what was happening in my body while I watched the swallows dip and dive, and particularly the sensations of the one flying circles around me.

I was filled with a sense of renewal and joy. One would think "out of nowhere", but it wasn't. It was from these birds, and the sensation of watching them, and, it seemed, something they were bringing me. I felt *included* in Life in a beautiful and unusual way.

Of Course, Nature Heals

I consciously let myself have a vicarious flight with the swallows, feeling the freedom in their bodies, and how whole they were. And, for some moments, these little birds soothed the pain in my body.

Was I making it up? Perhaps. But, I guess I'd say, who cares? Does it really matter whether the healing comes from the birds, Nature, or from my conscious (or imagined) connection to them? Or all those things? Because I felt better. My body felt better. My soul felt eased.

That's a lot when you're in pain.

Do birds have healing power, or Nature as a whole? Now that I ask that question, it almost seems silly to doubt it.

We are Nature too, and I think our nervous systems were made for being closer to the earth, walking barefoot on it, sleeping out under the stars, breathing fresh air, listening to bird song, and watching the movements of animals and letting that inform our own bodies.

And I think we have discounted the impact that not being close to Nature has on our bodies and our pain levels. I've asked this question before: are we creating more pain in our bodies on the whole (especially inexplicable pain) because we have forced our nervous system to conform to unnatural rhythms, cut off from its natural regulator (Nature) and a very real, visceral connection with the natural world?

On A Path to Well Being

Today, I felt like I got an answer. My body felt refreshed and energized, my pain levels soothed, and I had a much better sense of well being just from standing there in the morning sun and letting myself become fully aware, breathe in, and appreciate the offering from the swallows.

A Native American friend and teacher healed her cancer many years ago by spending weeks sitting for hours every day under a waterfall in Brazil, letting the natural force of the water wash everything away, including all the grief and sadness of her life, which she allowed to freely flow from her into the water.

Why not?

Tomorrow, I think I'll drive to the woods and walk barefoot on the earth. Maybe I'll do an experiment with pain levels and the amount of time I spend not only outside, but truly in tune with, listening to, and appreciating the movements, sounds, energies, and patterns of Nature.

Who knows? Maybe bird songs actually heal. Maybe dirt does. Maybe the sun is an elixir, and so is the moonlight if taken in with a kind of respectful, quiet, attuned and loving attention.

And maybe if those things don't completely heal, I will at least have a greater sense of well being along this road, and that's worth a lot too.

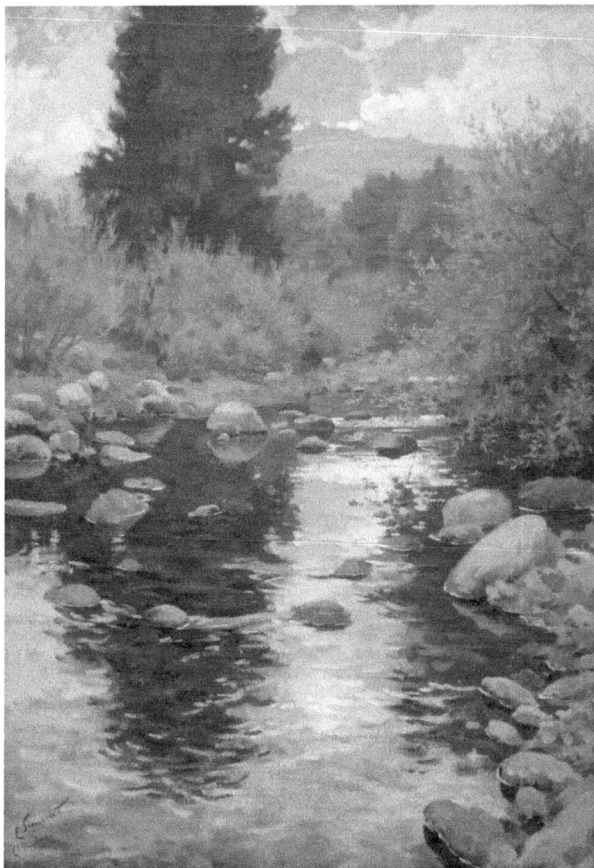

15

Making Our Journey

A Thing Of Beauty

I WATCHED A VIDEO of a tightrope walker recently, and my eyes welled up with tears because, as I watched his movements, I realized that they were such an illustration of life, and particularly, life with pain.

The man started walking along a tightrope suspended over a river and lost his balance. It looked like he would fall into the river, but he caught himself.

Then something absolutely wonderful happened.

He used the place of falling, the place that started to look like a mistake, started to look like failure, and made something new from it—something completely unexpected and creative. It was remarkably beautiful.

He used the falling motion as something chosen, something to play with and turn into another movement that was graceful and complete in itself. And he didn't fall completely, he turned, he twisted, he recalibrated, and restored his balance. And he did it again and again, using the rope not as a restriction but as a creative springboard.

The Way Across

I found watching him to be a very visceral and emotional experience. YES! I thought, this is exactly how we can be with our pain. We can cling to it, we can hang ourselves from it, we can twist ourselves up inside it and stay stuck and caught in it, suspended over an abyss OR we can use it to create beauty.

The tightrope and our pain are alike in that they both set parameters around experience, but they can not fully determine who we are. They do not determine our response. We may be living with severe limits, but we can create something new in that, through that, with that, and beyond that.

The tightrope limits, yes, but it is also a way across.

Pain limits, yes, but, somehow, it is also a way *to* something.

We may have to live with pain for a long time—we may have to keep coming back to it, just as the tightrope walker kept bouncing off and coming back to the rope—but we can also create a kind of awesome flexibility and resilience within that.

Using The Space Above And Around Pain

The tightrope walker could have had a stressful walk, focusing almost exclusively on his footing and the tightrope itself, trying to control every aspect of the experience the way we often focus on and try to control our pain experience.

Instead, through the looseness engendered by his fall,

his relationship to the tightrope becomes meaningful, alive, exuberant, and full of freedom. He shifts his focus to the spaces above and around the tight rope and uses it to propel him into places he never would have gone before.

And this is the way we can be with our pain, I feel.

Yes, we are in it, yes, it defines a lot about our lives, but we have choices within that and around that.

We can choose to focus on the pain itself as something to be overcome or eradicated or fought against. We can look down at it, metaphorically speaking, and hate it. We can stand in one place, our feet aching, our body tense, trying to hold our balance in one stuck position, whatever that may mean for us.

Or we can create.

Even with the pain, we can create. Even if our creativity is more internal than external, we can breathe, flex, adjust. We can re-learn to believe in ourselves and to dream.

Finding Places of Unexpected Beauty

Imagine if the tightrope walker had chosen to fight the rope, or cut it, or simply sit down and hang onto it. These are all options open to him, but look what he would have lost!

He completely changes his relationship not only to the rope but to the elements around it and the potentials they bring–he becomes more engaged with the air, with gravity, with his own body, and through this engagement he allows himself more freedom, and allows whatever happens to simply and elegantly inform his next move.

This is how we want to be with our pain, I believe.

We can imagine ourselves moving more freely, practicing inner agility, and creating a relationship with pain that is fluid, has breath, and may even propel us into unexpected places of freedom and beauty.

Headway by Access Oneness, www.yeahdude.fr direct video link: https://vimeo.com/147365891

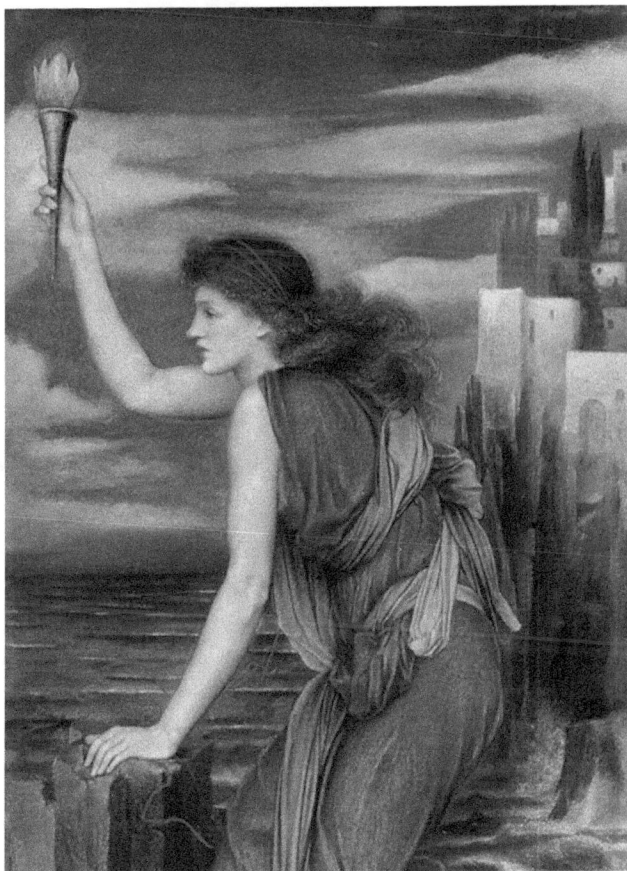

16

Losing And Finding

Ourselves in Pain

CHRONIC PAIN DISTANCES us from others, and, seemingly, from life itself. We are immersed within, and surrounded by, the experience of pain.

Everything other than pain recedes, and feels like it is being experienced from afar because there is always this aura of pain that separates us from others, and from life.

It's not that we're not in life, obviously we are still alive, but the quality of life is so different - as if we are looking out at life or up at life from a deeply submerged place.

Living Submerged

Other people exist on another plane. They have access to their bodies and their energy and their abilities while we are living underneath or within something. Sometimes it feels heavy, or dense, or foggy, or filmy. It can feel like living in a tank, and we must hear and see everything filtered through the thick glass and cloudy water.

When we live in pain for some time, it can begin to feel as if we are distanced not only from others and the ongoing stream of normal life, but from ourselves as well.

It is almost as if the field of pain has inserted itself between us and Us.

It's an eerie and unsettling feeling, kind of like when you have the flu or are terribly jet lagged and you don't feel like yourself–there is a sense of fogginess and existing apart from normal life and there isn't that much of You available.

The Cauldron of the Self

Living with chronic pain kind of feels like that all the time, and many times over. You fear you may have lost yourself in the pain. Or become someone else.

And there is a fear that you may never resurface, may never emerge from pain. And if and when you do, you won't know who you are anymore.

All of this can be incredibly frightening and depressing and sad, but there is also a strange gift here too.

Living submerged in pain can be like living in a cauldron or a furnace of the Self. It burns away everything that doesn't matter. It strips the self of everything petty and leaves only the essential Self that continues to shine.

You fear you will lose yourself, and in a way, you do lose yourself, or I should say, you lose the self that used to relate to the world in certain ways.

But you don't lose the inner Self.

Once you get past the fears and find a way to live with what is happening, to accept without giving up or acquiescing through allowing what's already here to be here as it is, the old you slides away, but you are not left with nothing. What's left is the essential Self, what I like to call the You of you.

Polishing The Mirror

None of this happens automatically as far as I can tell. We have a choice. We can become bitter and hardened, or we can choose to allow ourselves to be opened and enriched.

It's similar to what a former Sufi teacher of mine called "polishing the mirror". The challenges and hardships of life, if we meet them with awareness and allow them to show us what is essential and what is not, polish the mirror of the heart and allow the dross to drop away, and we are left with a clearer knowing of the Self.

And that Self is tender and vulnerable because of what it has been through, yes, but it's also incredibly strong.

You might call it your soul or spirit. It's the eternal aspect of you that remains alive and clear and untouched. And, while pain is a very difficult mentor and not one I would ever recommend to anyone, still, it teaches.

It brings us to our knees at times, but it also brings us to ourselves. And that, in its way, is a tremendous awakening and a tremendous gift.

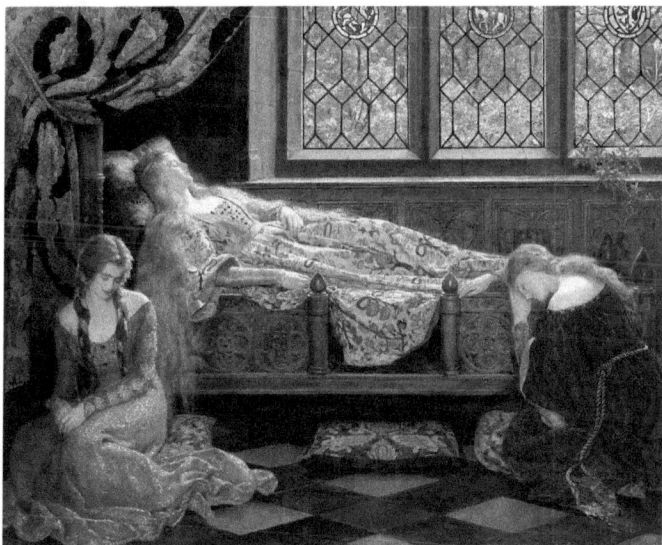

17

The Stories We Tell

COMING TO GRIPS with the fact that we're living in long-term pain can be incredibly challenging and distressing. To help make sense of it, we tell ourselves stories about what it all means.

That's not a bad thing if it gets us through another day. But sometimes we get stuck in our story and can't get to the next step or level in healing. Getting stuck can make us think there may not *be* a next step, or a next *anything*.

Here are some of the common tales we tell, and thoughts on how to get unstuck when they stop serving their purpose.

It's Only A Flesh Wound

This is often the first story we tell ourselves, sometimes even when we're in pretty dire straits. It's extremely hard to accept a severe or long-term illness or injury as a reality, and we feel that if we let that truth in, we will be letting the pain win. We'll be making it more real.

But we can't stay in denial forever if we want to move on in life. We have to face our situation head on, even if it means accepting the fact that moving forward means we are moving forward *with* pain for a time. Maybe a long time.

Keep My Seat, I'll Be Right Back

This is another flavor of denial that we often adopt once we've accepted that maybe whatever we're dealing with is more than a "flesh wound." So, we tell ourselves that it may look bad, but it will be over soon. Not a terrible thing to believe, of course–it's a way of staying positive.

On the other hand, if we sit in this story overly long, we may be avoiding some things we really need to deal with: That life has changed, that we may need to make some accommodations for the pain we're living with, that we may have to look at how pain is affecting our work life and our relationships over the long haul.

We may also be ignoring medical or alternative approaches that could really help us because we're choosing the story that we're not going to be doing this for long so there's no need to develop a long-term plan for living with pain.

It's kind of a tricky business–how to create a story that is both positive and realistic at the same time. We want to believe there's hope for moving beyond this soon, at the same time that we need to avoid ignoring the hard realities we have to be deal with right now.

The Answer Is Just Around The Corner

This story is about the belief that there is one final all-encompassing miracle cure to find and then everything will be all right.

When we tell ourselves this tale, we could be missing out on all the small, but important, things we can do right now to increase our well being because we're absorbed with searching for the one true answer. These small but important things include: Resting often, drinking lots of water, eating healthfully, laughing more, staying as stress free as possible, staying connected with friends, journaling or making music or dancing to express what we are going through and not letting it pool up inside.

We don't have to let go of hope for new developments and possibilities on the horizon, of course, but we also want to remember that healing is an everyday kind of thing that often happens in small increments over time.

There Is No Answer

This is the story we tell ourselves when we're discouraged. When we haven't found the answer after months and years of searching. We might decide that there really isn't *any* answer at all for us, and that we are lost in our pain forever. We might then conclude that we just have to live with the pain in a state of resignation. We lose hope and stop moving toward answers and start to dig in for the long haul.

This is when we need to remind ourselves again that there is probably no single answer to chronic pain, that the answer is—no matter how hard this can be to accept and live with—what we are living day by day. Our life has to *become* the answer, even as we keep open to new possibilities for recovering more of our functionality and more of ourselves as we move forward in life.

Pain Is Bigger Than Me

Another common tale is that pain is bigger than we are. It is so all encompassing, so demanding, and so ever-present that it can begin to feel like it has taken over our whole world.

We want to be careful not to confuse ourselves with our pain. Yes, it may be everywhere we go right now, but it is not the totality of who we are.

We need to remember to find ways to experience pleasures and joys alongside our pain whenever we can. Pain is an unpleasant experience we're having, but it is *within* our experience of life. It is not *all* of life or all of us.

Stories That Heal

Sometimes the story we tell ourselves is the only way to get up in the morning or to make it through the day, but sometimes the story is what's keeping us stuck.

I guess the question to ask is, how is my pain story serving me? Is there something I can change in it that will lead to a greater sense of hope, well-being, and renewal? Then we can choose to create a different tale to tell ourselves.

Maybe it becomes the story of how healing isn't some unknown point in the future, dependent upon one right answer, but what we do everyday. It becomes the story of finding ourselves again when we thought we were lost in the pain, and the story of allowing our healing to take the time it needs while maintaining the balance between acceptance of our current limitations and positive action toward a less painful future.

It becomes a story that focuses more on what we can do right now and where we're headed than about how we haven't healed yet and what hasn't worked. It becomes a story about courage, fortitude, creativity and quiet perseverance.

And it's a story we're free to modify, enlarge, or swap out as soon as it becomes outdated or restrictive.

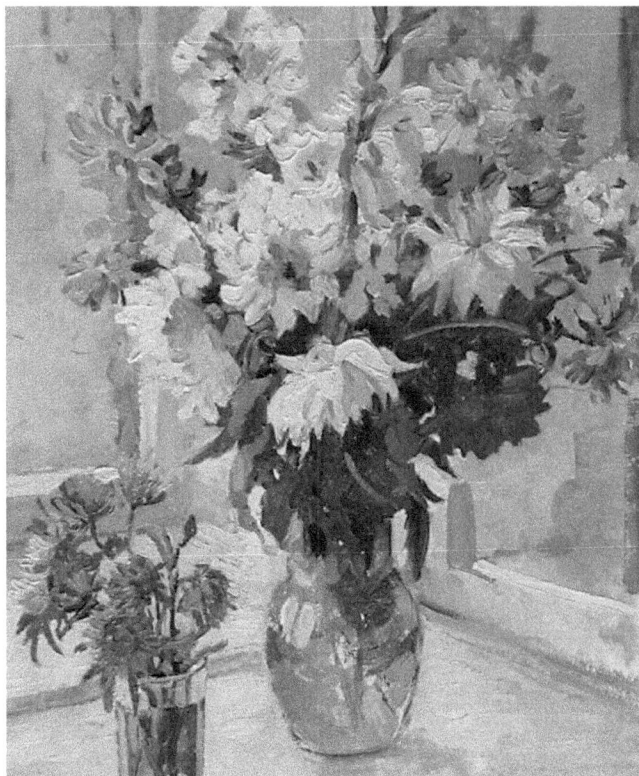

18

Writing Through Pain To See Myself

I'M FROM NEW ENGLAND, so the first answer I came up with for living with chronic pain was to grit my teeth and stoically carry on. Just live through it from day to day with as much grace and as little sourness as I could manage.

After several years of that, I thought, okay, I've been a good girl. I've slogged through my days as positively as possible with hardly any complaining and I've done everything within my capacity to heal.

So, why isn't the pain going away? This just can't be it. I can't live the rest of my life like this.

The Plan: Write Out The Pain

I had used journaling in the past to move through emotional challenges, so I thought, well, maybe I can *write* the pain out of my body.

Not very scientific, I know, but I was desperate.

Very slowly and very painfully I started writing a few sentences at a time about what it feels like to live with pain.

About how pain moves in and takes over your life. About how I hated the pain in my body. About all the things I was forced to give up and the time lost to pain. I wrote scathing letters to pain, demanding to know what it thought it was doing by taking up unpaid lodgings in my body.

After several months of this I noticed something. I noticed that I felt better. I couldn't say I'd cured myself, or that pain had left my body, not at all, but I felt better. *Despite* and *in* the pain. Huh.

Seeing Myself in the Pages

So I kept going. Over a couple of years of writing sentence by painful sentence with large rests between, sometimes lasting several months, I filled a couple of notebooks with spider scrawl. Then I stopped, read them, and saw what I'd been through.

First, I saw the terrible pain, the loss, the grief, and the hopelessness. I saw how chronic pain had robbed me of precious activities with my son, my work-related aspirations, and my avocations.

And that was very, very difficult to acknowledge and very sad, but it was also important to *see* the whole story. To witness myself, in a sense.

But, along with the many challenges, I also saw phenomenal strength, and a growing wisdom. I saw an absolute love for myself and for my son and for life, and the incredible tenacity of spirit that kept me going day after day.

And that was equally important to see and acknowledge and own.

What Pain Couldn't Take

So I wrote about my path with pain and through pain and saw myself in the writing. Not because I had *become* pain or because pain had overwhelmed who I was, but because, despite everything, *I* was still there.

Whole and complete.

The me of me was still intact. I had been through the fire, and what was left was pure me.

That was the beginning of healing–to write honestly and deeply about my experiences and to recognize that pain couldn't rob me of everything. It could rob me of a lot, but it couldn't rob me of myself.

Maybe that seems like a small jewel to dig out of the muck, but I really don't think so.

I know who I am. I know what I can go through. I know how strong I am and how much I can love. I know compassion and caring and softness and resilience.

And that's a lot. That's a lot.

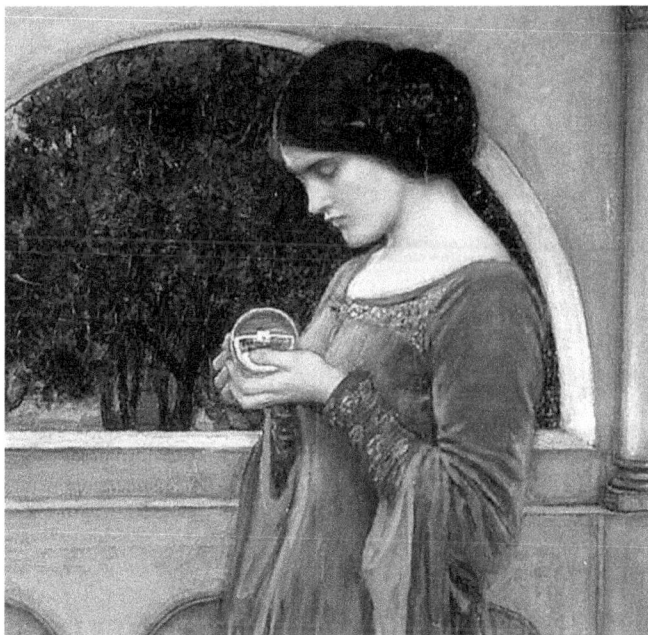

19

When Magical Thinking

Is Not Enough

WHILE THE NEW AGE movement certainly has at its core a plethora of valuable ideas that can help humanity, some of these ideas are not always entirely supportive of those of us in chronic pain– at least not at the superficial level most often touted by the movement's evangelists and motivational speakers.

We are lead to believe that if we can only think positively enough, visualize enough, and do enough affirmations, we will end our pain. That's the way it's supposed to work. Right?

Clap Your Hands And Believe

Um…well…

When I contracted my painful condition I was working in a spiritual bookstore. I had a library of metaphysical books on my own shelves at home, and all of them were well read from cover to cover. I could meditate, visualize, create intentions, and do affirmations with the best of them.

These techniques had all been wonderful boons at various times and helped me create loads of great experiences. But…

None of these things helped my pain once I was injured.

Not one.

And, because New Age magical thinking says you can change anything and this belief is becoming part of our collective consciousness, those of us who live with conditions that simply don't improve often feel like we've screwed up somehow. Why isn't it working for us?

Nice Ideas...For Some

So let's look at two main tenets of the New Age which are becoming more and more popular and, therefore, increasingly part of our collective ideas about reality:

1) If you think positively you can have anything you want.

2) Sickness and pain result from negativity and/or denial of Spirit.

Okay. Guess what? These principles may be fairly useless when you're in deep pain. Or, let's put it differently. These ideas may have some truth in them, but neither of them are the *whole* truth.

1) If You Think Positively, You Can Have Anything: It's a nice thought, and I do believe in being as positive as possible, I just haven't seen positive

thinking and affirmations work as a sweeping cure-all solution for chronic pain.

I'm all for thinking positively, just don't tell me I'm in pain because I'm not doing enough of it. For those of us who find ourselves living with physical pain, thinking positively is exhausting. It's really hard to get fired up with positive thoughts when you can barely stay in your body.

I don't know how any of the top New Age gurus would fare if they were plunked down in the middle of my life at the worst of my pain. It's incredibly challenging just to live through it, let alone drum up some magically enhanced enthusiasm.

Maybe the problem is not that we're doing it wrong, it's just that thinking positively for someone in chronic pain looks different than for someone whose body works.

Positive thinking for someone in chronic pain doesn't look like leaping through fields of daisies. It looks like getting out of bed and taking care of ourselves in small ways. Making a cup of tea. Eating well. Taking a short walk. Making one important phone call. It looks like deciding to keep going another day with as much dignity as we can muster.

2) All Pain is the Result of Negativity and/or Denial of Spirit: Most of us in pain go through times when

we're angry with Spirit, God, Creator, or whatever term we use for the divine being, but it doesn't mean we're in complete denial of our spiritual selves.

Many of us have had to find a way to get closer than ever to the spiritual aspects of Self and Life in order to carry on. We have had to dig more deeply, believe more strongly, and pull up more faith and hope from within the depths of ourselves to get through one more day than many people need in a year.

You're On A Different Path

I want to be clear here. I am not proclaiming that all New Age thinking and methods are useless. Not at all. My point here is, if you're in so much pain that you can't focus, or if the alternative methods don't work for you because your condition is so acute, or unusual, or recalcitrant in other ways, it does not mean you haven't tried hard enough. It's not your fault. It is a report card on these methods in relationship to your condition, not a report card on you.

So, it seems to me, that while New Age positive and magical thinking is great sometimes, it's simply not the whole story. It doesn't include the fact that sometimes we're in a situation for reasons that our rational mind, our everyday consciousness, just can't grasp.

And, try as we might to "positive" ourselves out of it, it does seem that some of us are simply on a part of our journey that includes pain, and, even though it's incredibly challenging, it's not our mistake.

As with the journey through grief, or the journey through birthing a baby, ours is a journey that also includes a level of deep pain for the time being. But that does not make it any less sacred, less true, or less valid than any other path. And it doesn't mean we're not being positive enough or spiritual enough.

Because, as far as I can see, healing chronic pain is not about trying to magic it away. It's not so much about constantly seeking a way to get around it, as it is living with as much grace as possible while living *through* it and all the way out to the other side.

And that is a deeply spiritual journey that requires true courage, an amazing amount of resilience, and a positive renewal of self on a daily basis.

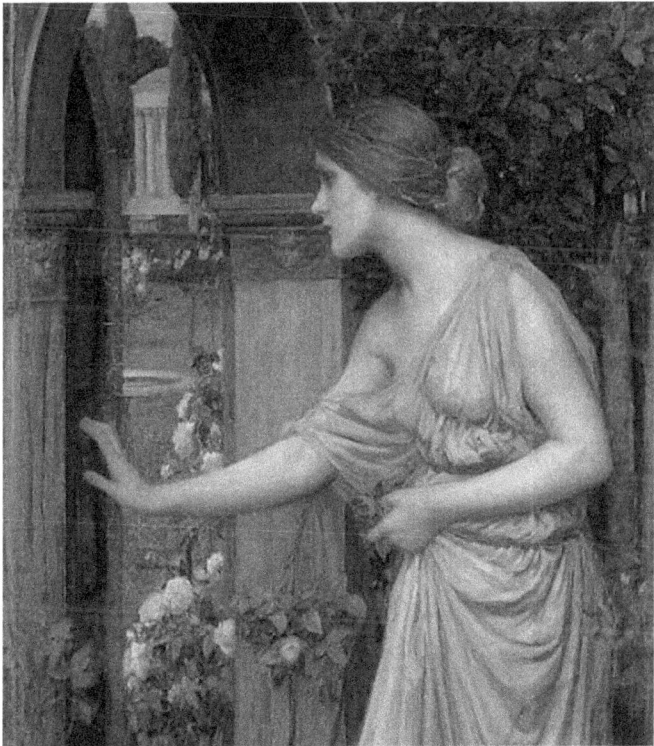

20

Truth As A Door To Deep Healing

THERE IS A MOMENT when you realize that your pain just isn't leaving. It has morphed from simple pain to chronic pain.

You may remember that moment very well. I certainly do.

I was driving down the road after a doctor's appointment in which I was informed that my Thoracic Outlet Syndrome was not getting any better, that I would most probably have it for the rest of my life, and that, in fact, it was most likely going to get progressively worse.

The Awful Truth

It was about a year into my pain journey. I had heard the doctor quite clearly, but it didn't really land until I was driving home. And then it hit me hard. A sort of cold, icy feeling in the middle of my chest.

Oh, I see, this isn't going away any time soon. Or in the vernacular: *I am really screwed.*

And even though I had been living with pain 24/7 for the past year, I just kept thinking it was about to leave. I had always healed from things in the past.

Nothing had ever stuck around this long. Any day now it was going to lift and just disappear.

Except it hadn't. And it wasn't going to, apparently.

And I finally let that in.

I felt depressed, lost, desolate, and hopeless for a while. I mean, what are you supposed to do with that kind of news? There's only so much positivity and hopefulness you can muster up to deal with an authoritative statement like that.

Accepting What's True

I didn't want to hear it, I didn't want to know it, I didn't want it to be real. Part of me wanted to blame the doctor for having ever said it, because saying it somehow made it more true.

And, certainly, a doctor's prognosis carries a lot of weight and does influence our ability to keep going, to keep a positive attitude, and to believe in ourselves and our ability to heal.

On the other hand, I'm grateful to have been told the truth. I now realize that the moment in the car when I allowed myself to accept the truth of my situation was probably the first step toward deep healing.

I had to accept that life had changed. Instead of assuming I was just going to get better by default, because that's what always happened in the past, I had to come to grips with the fact that I had a condition that didn't benefit by pretending it wasn't all that bad.

I needed to make some lifestyle changes, some accommodations, so that I didn't keep causing myself more pain by trying to force myself to keep up in ways that really weren't healthy for me.

I had to learn to simplify, to say no, and to take care of myself in new ways.

And that was hard.

Our Strange, Difficult, Beautiful Journey

But accepting what was true meant I could make more sane choices about what to say yes to and what to say no to.

It helped me take a longer view on healing and decide what I needed to do that would help me improve over time.

Instead of looking either for a non-existent quick fix, or simply trying to ignore the fact that my body was crying out for help, I had to take serious stock and make some decisions about how I was going to live and heal and ultimately thrive over the long run.

And these choices not only had positive effects on my pain levels, they enriched my life. Because slowing down, getting simple, taking it easy, and learning to say yes and no in appropriate ways taught me a lot about honoring myself and my path.

Coming to grips with the fact that I was living not just with pain, but with chronic pain was a thoroughly unpleasant realization to have, and I deeply commiserate with those of you who have had to come to that moment.

But it was also a very important moment, and a key to beginning to heal on deeper levels.

What a strange, difficult, and oddly beautiful journey we're on, those of us in chronic pain.

Some of the most difficult times of having to face pain, accept it, and just be with it have the potential to also become doors to deep healing and transformation.

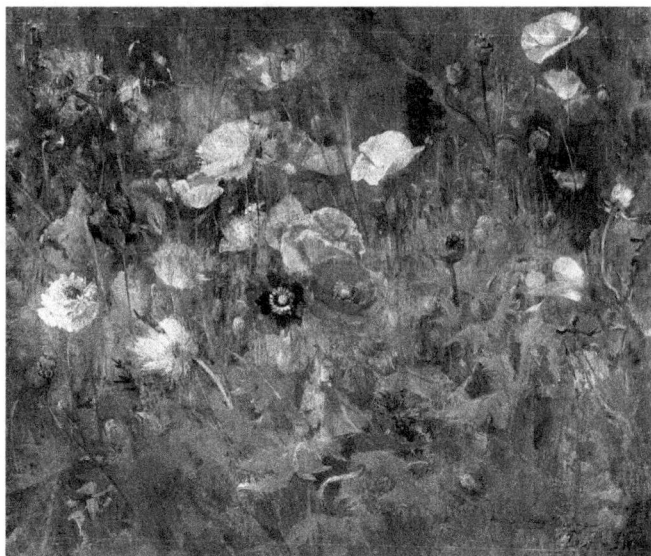

21

Is Pain Pointing Toward Life?

I GOT UP THIS MORNING after one of *those* nights. You know. When you shift around trying to get comfortable but each new position feels worse than the last.

Anyway, I guess it made me feel philosophical about pain and pain's purpose, and what this is all about.

And I thought, what if pain is the only way we'll slow down enough to really take a good look at ourselves and at our lives?

The Unseen Hand

I mean, what if, in a sense, pain is the hand that pulls us back from some dangerous precipice? It's uncomfortable, sudden, and shocking even, but maybe it's actually saving our lives in some unknown manner.

If we look at where pain forces us to go, what it forces us to do, then maybe it makes some sense. Pain asks us to look inward, to be in the body, to live in the moment, to take stock, to re-prioritize, to slow down, to let go, to simplify.

These are mostly pretty healthy things to do.

Are they things we would have done anyway? Possibly not. Certainly, I wouldn't have. I resent the fact that pain forced me to do these things, and I would prefer to have chosen them on my own, but I didn't.

I'd Like a Renewal, Please

So, is pain pointing us toward a renewal of spirit, a renewal of life?

This might seem to imply that we made a mistake, or did something wrong to get into pain in the first place. But I don't like to think of it that way.

If I've learned anything from my time in pain, it's that self-blame and self-recrimination are not useful, necessary, or accurate stances to take toward the self.

Maybe then, pain is a kind of course adjustment.

To me, the beginning of pain feels like a strong contraction away from something, like the area in pain has become a fist tightly closed, or a black hole pulling inward and away–a massive retraction as a reaction to the pain. It is a pulling away from the sensation of pain, but also a retraction from life.

Thinking of it this way, pain is more of an absence than a presence.

What if pain is the sensation of something missing or lost? Well, yes, you say, health is missing, of course, but what is health but a full engagement with life?

How Does Pain Ask Us To Change?

So, it seems that part of healing is the re-engagement with life, a re-engagement coming from a new stance within the self after having gone through the massive contraction from life that was apparently necessary for some reason (perhaps only the soul knows why.)

So, the questions become—what does pain ask of us, and what are we asking of ourselves to change, to embrace, to move toward in order to heal?

How is pain pointing us toward life?

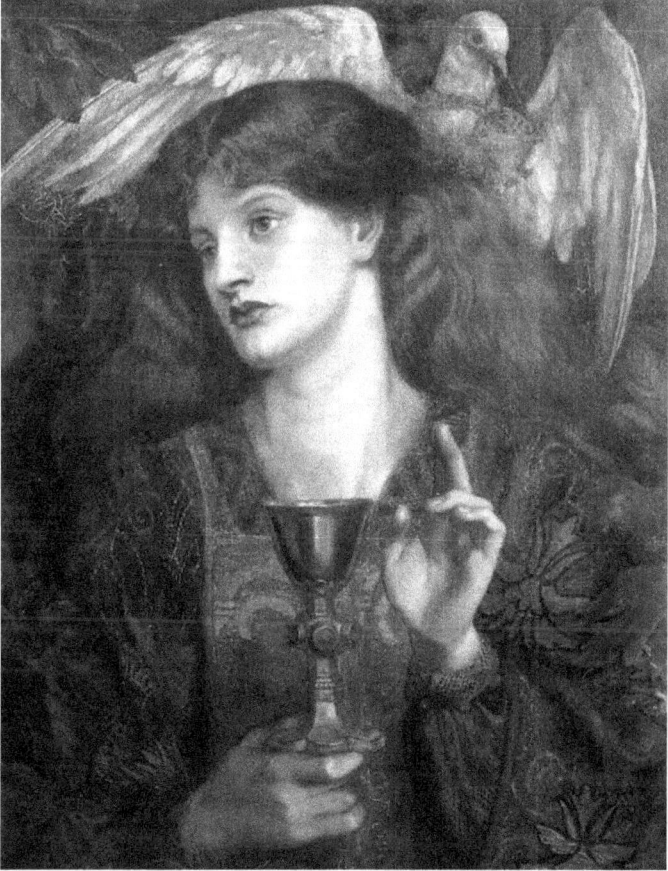

22

The Myth of the Holy Grail of Pain

OUR MODERN CULTURE excels in building up an expectation of right answers for everything. We are put through years and years of schooling with all manner of exams and tests that imply that there is an answer for every question.

Not only does an answer exist, but there is only one correct answer and all the rest are wrong, even if they're really, really close.

It Must Be Out There Somewhere

So, we've had it trained into us to believe that everything, everything, everything must have a solution, and the solution is singular.

It must be out there somewhere. We just haven't found it yet.

We imagine that if there were a teacher's report of our lives, it has red marks all over it to show where we've screwed up because we haven't found the perfect fit, or the perfect key, or the perfect response to life.

And this carries over to the way we are with ourselves in pain and the way we respond to life with pain.

We search for the real fix, the magic pill, the one true key to healing, to a pain free existence, to a more satisfying life. Or even one that is just slightly less painful than the one we have now.

There must be *an* answer to chronic pain. What is it? Where is it? Who has it? So we keep searching the pharmaceutical shelves, the internet, the medical community, and within ourselves.

Where Have I Gone Wrong?

What have I done wrong? we ask ourselves over and over. Where haven't I looked, because I don't have that one answer yet, and I *know* that there has to be a right answer out there somewhere.

We go from being determined to find it, to being frustrated with the last thing we tried that didn't work, to panicking that we will never find the answer we're looking for, to being despondent, and, finally, defeated. (And then, after a period of despondency, we usually find a way to pick ourselves up and start that cycle over again.)

We may feel our doctors have failed us. We may feel life has failed us. We may feel we have failed at life. We may feel we have failed ourselves, failed at *being* ourselves in this life because this isn't what we signed up for.

So we keep looking for the holy grail for pain.

It's out there, somewhere, it must be. Because that's the way the world is set up, isn't it? That's what was drilled into us for years and years and years, that there is an answer to every question, a singular answer, so we can't stop searching for that grail.

Every day we put on our suit of armor and continue the quest. And we often exhaust ourselves with the search.

The Answer is Not Singular

But perhaps there isn't only one true answer for persistent pain, just like there isn't only one valid path through life. The answer may not be in one pill, one procedure, one supplement, one alternative treatment, and it may not happen on one specific day.

The answer does not, in fact, appear to be singular at all.

Long-lived pain seems to require a multi-layered and complex series of responses that draw input from all aspects of the self.

And maybe that seems discouraging, that there may not be one final pill, or one all-encompassing treatment for our long-lived pain. But I don't think so. I think it can also be a kind of relief.

Instead of making ourselves wrong for not having found the one true answer, the holy grail for pain, we can know that everything we do with an intention to heal *is* part of the answer, That we are, in fact, already living the answer with every breath we take .

The answer is not a state of absolute correctness, a final knowing that will set everything right all at once.

Instead, it seems to be a messy, many-faceted, imperfect, and ever-changing process made up of the best choices and responses we can manage from one day to the next, and which may include many approaches and many methods over time.

So, Do We Give Up The Search?

There may not be a mythical shining chalice we have to keep believing in that we need to set out in search of. Instead, the answers may be closer than we think, right here with us. Not something elusive and unobtainable, but something we make for ourselves. Something we *live*.

Does that mean that we should stop looking for answers to chronic pain? Not at all.

But I do believe that if we haven't found the one true solution yet, it may be that is isn't in just *one* place, it may be that we are surrounded by pieces of the holy grail, so to speak.

Each of these pieces, taken together, can create a workable approach for us made up of daily choices—

some of which may be choices we revisit that didn't help before and now do, some may be from other disciplines and not strictly medical in flavor, and some may be new medical developments.

So, we fashion our own grail that reflects who we are and what we need as we move through our journey with pain, and, instead of being something we have to find, it is something we create for ourselves through our choices and through our quest for wholeness.

The shape and size and design of the grail may shift and change from day to day as we adapt our healing path to the way our condition unfolds, but we stay responsive and open to new means and renewed hope because the most hopeful answer we have is that our answer is not one, but many.

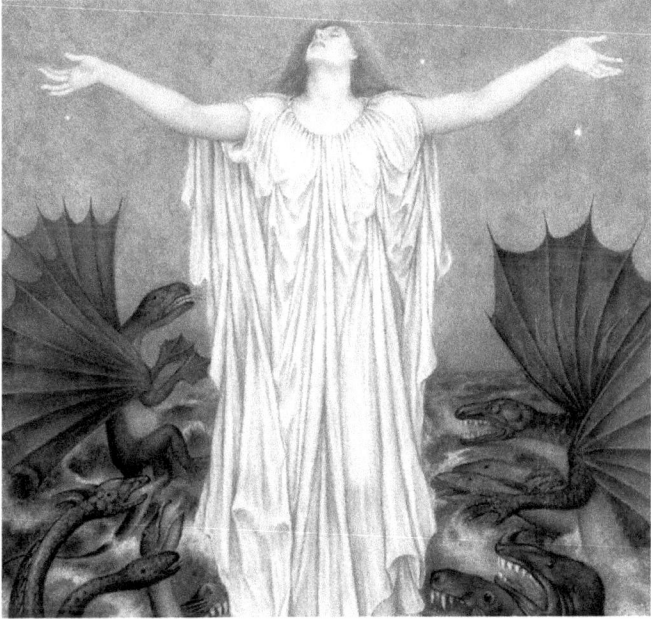

23

A Different Kind of Animal

ONE OF THE REASONS we may not be healing from chronic pain is that we are expecting the ongoing pain that we are experiencing now to act like the pains we have suffered in the past.

We anticipate that all pain will become noticeably less acute as time passes and, eventually to lose its sting. That's what happens when you stub your toe. That's what happens when you burn your hand. That's even what happens when you grieve a loss.

It Won't Ride Off Into The Sunset

The other pains in life may be small, they may be huge, they may be overwhelming, but they all have a time frame. They arrive, we experience them in their smallness or bigness, and they quickly or slowly fade away. But they do fade away.

If not completely, then enough that we can move on with life and at some point in the future we realize that we don't hurt any more in that way. The pain fades into the distance, as if it is linked to time as it recedes into the past.

The problem with the way we are thinking about and treating chronic pain is simply that it isn't the same *kind* of pain. We tend to address chronic pain with treatments created for short-term pain, but, for the most part, it refuses to budge.

Of course, chronic pain shows up initially as if it is like all other physical pains. It is not chronic yet, it is simply pain. So, naturally, we begin by treating it like any other pain. But there comes a point when we have to recognize that we're dealing with a different beast.

Time To Take A Different Road

This is when we have to reevaluate our strategy. After one or two or three months of persistent pain, we come to understand that the nature of the pain we are dealing with is simply not the same as short-term pain.

However, despite this re-labeling of our pain to chronic pain, most of the time we don't change our strategy. We continue further along the same road of treating all pain alike. We think that if we do more of the same things, or do them longer, then we're addressing chronic pain.

After a point, however, it becomes clear that there just doesn't seem to be any obvious healing for us down that road.

In addition, chronic pain comes with other physical ailments—or side effects—that don't always fall under the category of "pain", yet are, nevertheless, part of our experience of long-term pain. These include intense fatigue, inability to think clearly, constant flu-like symptoms, and an overall feeling of fogginess and depression, among others.

When we tell practitioners about our symptoms, they may stop us once we've described what falls into the normal "pain" category. They don't always want to know about the rest, either because they don't consider fatigue, overwhelm, fogginess, or depression as part of the "pain package" or because they simply don't know what to do about them. As a result, we are often left feeling misunderstood and unheard.

Not All Pain Is The Same

For all these reasons, I feel it is important that we begin to think of chronic pain not just as pain that sticks around, but as a different *kind* of pain altogether. It is in its own category and requires its own approach to healing.

Too often, when medical practitioners feel stymied by chronic pain, they tend to blame the sufferer or disbelieve their reports of continued pain. Instead of blaming the patient, however, this should signal that our treatments, approaches, protocols and attitudes toward chronic pain need to be revamped, updated, and enlightened.

Since chronic pain eludes the efforts of our doctors to end it, we must understand that it therefore requires long-term treatment using a multi-layered approach, perhaps with many different practitioners.

We need to consider modalities, treatments, and approaches that do not just begin where short-term treatments leave off, but which look at, handle, and relate to pain in completely different ways right from the moment we realize our pain is chronic–ways that include the effects of chronic pain not only on the physical body, but on the emotions, psyche, and identity of the sufferer.

We need to understand that chronic pain is intrinsically a *unique condition* from short-term pain. It is dissimilar in the way it is generated, felt, experienced over time, and healed.

It is altogether a different kind of animal.

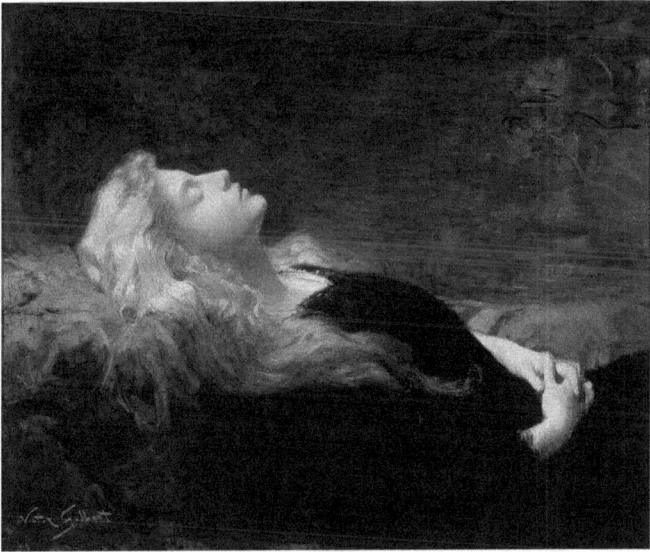

24

The Light at the Center of Pain

ANY KIND of long-lived pain eventually sinks into and penetrates to the deepest levels of the Self.

This deeper level is very intimate with the Soul and lies close to who we think we are. After living with pain for many months, it can feel like our pain becomes intertwined with and seemingly inseparable from us at the core of who we are, the core of our identities.

I have become this pain. This pain has become me.

Pain sends tendrils inward from surface experience, down, down, down into the center of the Self to grow roots there.

The Well Within

It's as if there is a deep well somewhere in all of us. It's part of being human. Most of us only dip into that well briefly when we meet life's challenges, difficulties, and losses, and then we (mostly) return to life as usual.

Some of us go wading in the depths of the well from time to time when we are doing some soul searching, and some of us end up immersed in it when we are depressed, unable to find our way out again because it seems that we are in a cistern with slippery sides and no footholds.

Once any pain has stayed and stayed and stayed, the experience can become one of submersion of the self–a forced immersion in the inner worlds to the bottom of that well because we feel we have lost most of our outer world and, ultimately, we are left with only ourselves. Just us with us.

What Chronic Pain Demands

I think that's part of what chronic pain is, somehow–or what it demands–a sinking into the deeper levels of the self to take a difficult and often dark journey to the core of who we are.

If we allow ourselves to follow the tendrils of pain inward and down, all the way to their roots and then not stop there, just keep going deeper and deeper (trying not to fight it too much), we may pass through our field, of pain, and if we keep going, we may find the essential self just beyond, fine and bright and clear as it has always been.

So it seems that, at least for some of us, the path to the core of the self requires us to go through the pain in order to reach the brightness at the center.

What We Bring Back

And I think we can pull something from the inner core, some light and some knowing, and travel back out with it, passing through the pain field again, but this time the pain is lessened, is not so penetrating.

We emerge back into our lives with something impossibly beautiful—some knowing, some understanding, some pure experience of our most true self—that is wise and dear and valuable.

It isn't the path we would have chosen for ourselves, and pain may still be there in our outer experience, but there is also the experience of this astonishingly clear and unexpectedly beautiful Center.

This wisdom, this knowing, this offering, is informed by pain, yes, but is not made entirely of pain. It has deepened and been strengthened by its journey *through* pain, and emerges clear and authentic, carrying a core of light at its center.

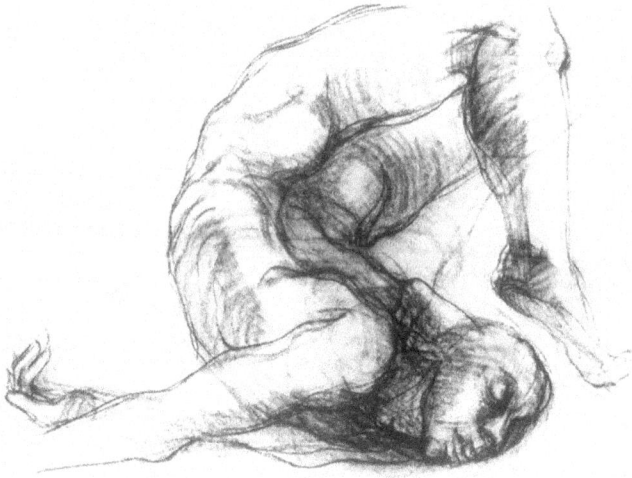

25

Making Peace With Pain

IT'S THAT TIME of year. We all do it. We make our list of New Year's resolutions.

Or we decide we're done with lists, and we're just going to choose the one thing we're really going to do this year.

And then, about three days later, we realize we've already forgotten what was on the list. Or that doing that one thing is going to be harder than we thought.

You're Not Lazy

It's not that we can never keep our promises to ourselves, or that we're undisciplined, or lazy, or bad people. It's because we usually choose things we *haven't been able to do yet* to go on that list of New Year's resolutions. And the reason we haven't been able to do them yet is because they're hard.

So, we start fresh on the 1st of January (or the 2nd or the 3rd), using the beginning of the calendar year to start a metaphoric new beginning in life.

And sometimes it works. Sometimes we get some good momentum going and we really do keep those resolutions.

But a lot of the time we don't. Not because we're awful people, but because if our resolutions were easy to keep, we would have done them already.

Last year.

But I Don't Want To Be In Pain This Year

And here we are in a new year, and we're still dealing with pain. It would be great to make a resolution for this year to be pain free, wouldn't it?

How do we do that? If we make a resolution to be pain free, if we put that on our list, we almost immediately feel a sense of futility. How can we make that happen? How can we commit to something over which we feel we have very little control?

In my experience, pain is the uncooperative factor in that resolution. It just won't be ordered around.

It's not that we aren't strong enough. It's that pain has it's own longevity, and its own purpose. We certainly may not understand what that is, but it seems to be so.

Pain will take the time it takes.

Let Go of Resolutions

So, this year, at any time, not just New Year's, a wonderful resolution would be to let go of resolutions and just be with what's in life right now, even if it includes pain.

We make a resolution to stop fighting the big battle. This isn't the same as giving up or giving in or giving over as if we're crawling into our pain and disappearing inside it. Not at all.

Giving up the battle with pain doesn't mean surrender, it means taking the energy we've been investing in resisting and fighting the situation and putting it into accepting that it's here now, and in finding ways to partner with pain and work with it as a messenger and a natural part of our healing path.

Why would we want to do that?

Because as long as we battle with pain, the battle will continue. When we stop clenching down on our pain, trying to stop it, and trying to fight it, it doesn't have to fight with *us* quite so much.

Paradoxically, when we allow pain the time it needs, when we stop resisting its presence, it seems to begin to complete it's mission faster.

Make Peace with Pain

Now maybe what I just wrote made you feel uncomfortable or angry with me. Maybe you think I don't understand how hard it is. But, believe me, I do. I do understand. It's relentlessly hard to live in pain.

But it's harder to keep struggling against it. Pain is

already here. And, so far, pushing against it hasn't made it go away.

So, as a scientific experiment, right now, take a moment to release your breath (are you holding it?). Let it flow naturally, and just allow the pain in your body to be what is, as it is, just for a moment.

Just for this moment, relax around the pain in your body. Allow pain to have the space it already occupies anyway.

It may be scary to you, and you may feel very vulnerable, but just for this moment, right now, don't fight with pain. It's still going to feel uncomfotable, but you're not fighting against it.

Notice You. And notice the pain. Coexisting. Making peace.

It's Not Weakness, Or Giving Up

So, consider making your next resolution a non-resolution. A resolution of letting go–releasing the battle with pain, and making peace with it starting with little intervals at a time–and watching what happens.

Being at peace with pain isn't a place of weakness or giving up. It's a place of great strength and, yes, even beauty.

LIST OF ILLUSTRATIONS

Luna, Evelyn de Morgan, 1885	1
Study, Evelyn de Morgan, date unknown	7
S.O.S., Evelyn de Morgan, (1914-16)	13
Resting, Victor Gabriel Gilbert, 1890	19
The Damsel of the Sanct Grael, Dante Rossetti, 1874	25
A Grecian Girl, John William Godward, 1908	33
Birches, Edge of the Forest, Isaac Levitan, 1878	39
The Answer, John William Godward, 1917	45
Dryad, Evelyn de Morgan (1884-5)	53
Ariadne in Naxos, Evelyn de Morgan (1877)	59
Lady Writing a Letter with Her Maid, Johannes Vermeer, 1670	65
Gather Ye Rosebuds, John William Waterhouse, 1909	71
Miranda, John William Waterhouse, 1875	77
In Realms of Fancy, John William Godward, 1911	85
Waldlandschaft, Alois Kirnig, (1840-1911)	91
The Belvedere, John William Godward, 1913	97
Swallow on Thorn Branch, Toshun, (1747-1797)	103
El Paular, Enrique Simonet, 1921	111
Hero Holding the Beacon for Leander, Evelyn de Morgan, 1885	117
The Sleeping Beauty, John Collier, 1921	125
Flowers, Tatiana Kopnina, 1957	131
The Crystal Ball, John William Waterhouse, 1902	137
Psyche Opening the Door Into Cupid's Garden, John William Waterhouse, 1903	145
A Bed Of Poppies, Maria Oakey Dewing, 1980	151
Circle Shape, Noella Roos Boris (date unknown)	157

ABOUT THE AUTHOR

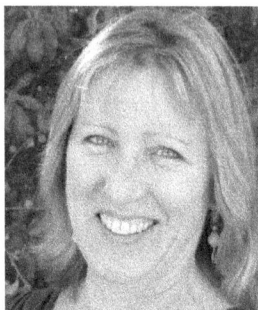

A native of Connecticut, Sarah Anne Shockley is a multiple award winning producer and director of educational films, including *Dancing From The Inside Out,* a highly acclaimed documentary on disabled dance. She holds an MBA in International Marketing and has worked in high-tech management, as a corporate trainer, and teaching undergraduate and graduate business administration. As the result of a work related injury in the Fall of 2007, Sarah contracted Thoracic Outlet Syndrome (TOS) and has lived with debilitating nerve pain since then. She is the author of *The Pain Companion*, and *Living Better While Living in Pain.* She resides in the San Francisco Bay Area.

Visit the author's website for free resources including *The Pain Companion Blog* and *The Pain Companion Oasis:* www.thepaincompanioncom.

OTHER BOOKS BY
SARAH ANNE SHOCKLEY

"Excellent resource. Great support."
-U. S. Pain Foundation

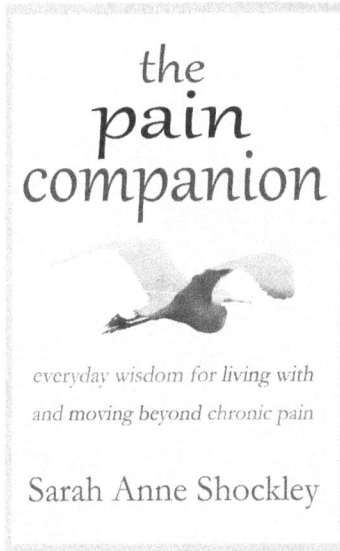

The Pain Companion: Everyday Wisdom for Living With & Moving Beyond Chronic Pain
Available in paperback, ebook, & audio formats

The Pain Companion is a practical guidebook to chronic pain management and chronic pain relief.
- create more ease and well being on a daily basis
- relieve the impact that living with pain has on well being, self-image and relationships
- alleviate pain's emotional, mental, and physical stresses

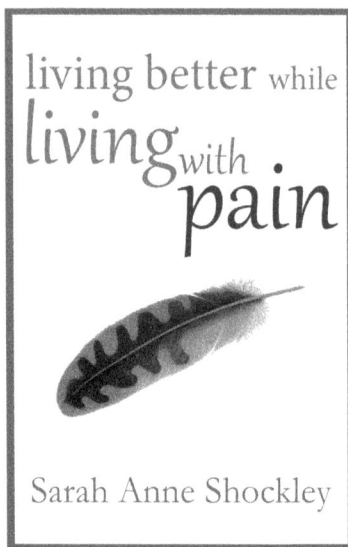

Living Better While Living With Pain
Available in print, ebook, & audio formats

A practical discussion of chronic pain, its differences from short-term pain, and suggestions for approaches to pain management and pain reduction specific to chronic pain. Includes 21 useful tips for creating more ease, comfort, and resiliency.

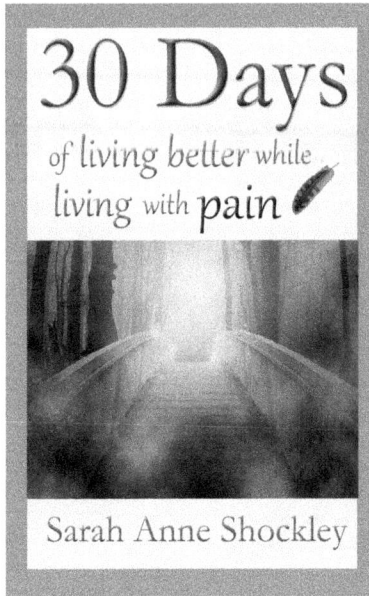

30 Days of Living Better While Living With Pain
Available in print & ebook formats

30 brief daily readings and images with suggestions and insights to relieve the emotional and spiritual stresses of living with chronic pain. Based on the author's popular book, *Living Better While Living With Pain.*

www.ingramcontent.com/pod-product-compliance
Lightning Source LLC
Chambersburg PA
CBHW060042030426
42334CB00019B/2441